SERVICE LINE

SUCCESS:

Eight Essential Rules

SERVICE LINE SUCCESS:

Eight Essential Rules

E. Preston Gee

ACHE Management Series

Health Administration Press

Your board, staff, or clients may also benefit from this book's insight. For more information on quantity discounts, contact the Health Administration Press Marketing Manager at (312) 424-9470.

08   07   06   05   04   5   4   3   2   1

Library of Congress Cataloging-in-Publication Data

Gee, Erin Preston.
    Service line success: eight essential rules / by E. Preston Gee.
      p. cm.
    Includes bibliographical references.
    ISBN 1-56793-217-7 (alk. paper)
    1. Health facilities—Administration. 2. Product management. 3. Hospitals—Marketing—Management. I. Title.

RA971.G39 2003
362.11'068'8—dc22

                                                2003061238

The paper used in this publication meets the minimum requirements of American National Standard for Information Sciences—Permanence of Paper for Printed Library Materials, ANSI Z39.48-1984. ∞ ™

Acquisitions manager: Audrey Kaufman; Project manager: Cami Cacciatore; Cover design: Betsey Perez; Layout editor: Amanda J. Karvelaitis

Health Administration Press
A division of the Foundation of the
    American College of Healthcare Executives
1 North Franklin Street, Suite 1700
Chicago, IL 60606-4425
(312) 424-2800

Contents

Preface

WAY BACK IN the mid-1980s my colleague, Jim Folger, and I coauthored a book for the American Hospital Association on an emerging concept in the healthcare field. The strategy was called product line management, or PLM. PLM had been attempted in many industries in the United States, achieving greatest prominence and success in the consumer goods field. Jim and I had both worked with consumer goods firms prior to migrating to healthcare administration. Jim had worked for the Heinz Corporation, and I had worked for Fisher-Price Toys, which at the time was a subsidiary of the Quaker Oats Company.

Our book was greeted with considerable interest and reasonable success—at least for a professional book in this field. A large number of hospitals throughout the country attempted, in one form or another, to incorporate product line precepts into their overall strategy. However, for whatever reason, the model was largely misunderstood and consequently misapplied. The outgrowth of all that misunderstanding was that PLM had a relatively short life span in its first introduction to healthcare.

Now fast forward to the early years of the twenty-first century: The industry is once again interested in the concept of service line (we have modified the name slightly) management, or SLM. The many reasons for this renewed interest will be discussed throughout the book. Whatever the cause for its current consideration, the fact remains that SLM is experiencing a resurgence in popularity, which is likely to surpass the exploration and implementation of the model in its first wave. I, for one, am encouraged and enthused about this revitalization of SLM for two reasons.

First, I think there is a more astute understanding of the true nature and application of SLM and its capacity to favorably position an organization within a competitive framework. Second, I think SLM has the potential to lift many healthcare organizations (hospitals and health systems) out of the economic doldrums and frustrating fluctuations that presently plague this industry, arguably to a greater degree than ever before.

For that reason, I am once again advocating SLM—a concept that has proven invaluable to myriad companies and multiple industries in the United States (and elsewhere) but has not (yet) taken root in healthcare. Perhaps this time around we will understand something our corporate colleagues have known for years: Service (or product) line management is not only sound strategy, it is also essential to long-term existence in a market-driven economy.

Chapter 1 makes the case for why a service line structure is the most strategic organizational design for competing in these turbulent times. Once that case has been made, the basic elements and essential components of service line management will be described in detail. Chapter 2 distills the formula down to eight essential rules that can be followed and instituted in almost any hospital or health system in the country. The reader is given the obvious option to tailor the application of these rules—detailed in chapters 3 through 10—to his or her particular organizational setting, but the fundamental framework is provided. The design of the model—service line structure—is such that it lends itself to ready implementation for a few key lines. In fact, that is what I suggest that managers consider in adopting the construct and incorporating the concept into the managerial design. Service line management means a thousand things to a thousand people, but giving it some defined parameters and probable objectives should help healthcare leaders better understand and apply its proven efficacy.

Acknowledgments

SO MANY INDIVIDUALS and organizations have provided practical information and valuable insight on this concept, and to that vast group I am indebted. Yet for the sake of brevity, I will only mention a few. First, I need to acknowledge the early-on collaboration of my friend and coauthor (of the original book on the subject) Jim Folger for his significant contributions to the product line/service line management model.

I would also like to recognize my professional colleagues at the St. David's Healthcare Partnership—especially Tom Coefield, who has provided many years of consistent encouragement and invaluable support. I also want to recognize the professional observations and contributions of my consulting colleague Frank Kittredge.

And finally (and most important) I want to acknowledge the tremendous support and encouragement of my wife, Janice, and our children—particularly our youngest son, Scott, to whom this book is dedicated.

CHAPTER 1

Second Time's the Charm

THIS FIRST CHAPTER gives a little background on the concept of service line management (SLM) and tells why the model is experiencing renewed popularity within the industry. The basis for its applicability and its proven success in other industries is also discussed.

WHY SERVICE LINE MANAGEMENT IS EXPERIENCING A RESURGENCE

The concept of service line management (known as product line management in the 1980s) is experiencing a major resurgence in the healthcare industry. The model was first launched in this industry in the mid-1980s, became popular through the early 1990s, and then went into a long dormancy period. Lately, however, hospital and health system executives are dusting off the idea and bringing it back into their organizations. Although there are many reasons for this, at the center of the movement is the tumult within the industry.

Healthcare in the United States is at a crossroads. With costs spiraling out of control and with the number of uninsured headed toward an all-time high, the clamor for solutions has never been more pronounced. Among these proposed solutions are two polarized options. At the end is to have consumers take a more active role in their healthcare—to have them more engaged, with more economic accountability and responsibility. At the opposite end of the spectrum is nationalized healthcare in one form or another.

Over the next few years there will likely be extensive debate on these options as well as the many alternatives in between. Either way the national debate goes, SLM provides an excellent framework for managing a healthcare organization. If the push is toward a consumer-driven model, SLM offers the optimal configuration for aligning with the consumer, because it originated in consumer-oriented industries. SLM employs the metrics of consumer-centric sectors with elements such as market research, strategic business units, portfolio analysis, and segmentation.

On the other hand, if the move is toward a universal or nationalized healthcare system, SLM enables an organization to identify inefficient service lines (which would be hindered by fixed payment) and isolate attention and resources on centers of excellence. A move toward a centralized system would occur gradually, and may (at least at the outset) involve a single-payer system of insurance. Under that scenario, just as with the government's move to the diagnosis-related group (DRG) system in the mid-1980s, SLM allows an organization to better understand the dynamics at play within the subcategories of its business. This understanding enables a hospital or health system to focus on the driving forces that determine the basis for success, in this case the reimbursement structure. SLM provides the framework for individual and organizational accountability, but it does so at a level where appropriate adjustments can be made in time to remedy quality concerns, minimize losses, and optimize organizational resources.

SLM PROVIDES MARKET FLEXIBILITY

The current configuration found in most hospitals does not allow for the flexibility required for these economically tenuous times.

In part, this is why so many facilities suffered financial difficulty following the first few years of DRG implementation and the Balanced Budget Act of 1997 (BBA). The financial, operational, and accountability structure of most hospitals simply does not foster ready and successful adaptation of a new delivery overlay. SLM enables an organization to better understand and implement such wide-scale changes.

The healthcare system—especially the hub of that system, which consists of hospitals and health systems—does not adjust well to major change. While this is understandable, it is neither admirable nor sustainable. Healthcare systems (and to a lesser extent, hospitals) are like supertankers: When faced with the need to change course as a result of external forces, or internal considerations, extensive time and considerable effort are necessary to implement that change. That metaphoric reality holds true for many, if not most, of the hospitals in the United States. If one does not believe that, then one should review the operational results of the majority of hospitals in the years following DRG implementation (1984, 1985, and 1986) and subsequent to BBA enactment (1998 and 1999). While one could argue that these two major events provided powerful and sweeping, as well as profound and pervasive, changes to the delivery system, some hospitals or systems did adjust, adapt, and emerge as operationally and financially viable as they did prior to these events—and did so in less than five years.

The Need to Be More Malleable to Market Dynamics

On average, however, most hospitals took a great deal of time to regain their operational and financial positions, thanks largely to eventual adjustments of the regulations and political pressure and intervention by outside agencies. Interestingly, most hospitals have still not regained the financial position they enjoyed prior to BBA enactment, as the average margins for hospitals across the nation are still lower than they were in 1996 (Health Care Advisory Board 2003).

This point is emphasized to underscore that monumental changes are a part of the healthcare landscape. The kind of sweeping change witnessed with the implementation of DRGs and the enactment of the BBA pales in comparison to the probable sea change that lies ahead in the very near future. Fundamentally, SLM offers the optimal configuration for dealing with such industrywide changes, as is evidenced by the performance of the past. At its core, SLM is a much more elegant and sophisticated configuration for dealing with this kind of change (or any other) because it enables an organization to rapidly assess its vulnerable areas and make the necessary adjustments.

The inherent beauty of the SLM structure is that it forces the organization to institute a discipline of measurement and accountability that exists in nearly every other industrial sector of American enterprise. Some leaders have balked at the need for such a structure, arguing that "We're not selling widgets or operating hotels." However, such provincial reasoning only highlights a misunderstanding of the basic precepts of SLM and obviates the considerable benefits of such a design. At its most rudimentary level, SLM is merely a subdividing of the organization into manageable, measurable, and accountable components.

A FUNDAMENTALLY MISUNDERSTOOD CONCEPT

Much of the failure in past application or implementation of SLM lies in the fundamental misunderstanding of the concept. During its first wave in the mid- to late 1980s, the model was misconstrued as primarily a marketing vehicle (this will be discussed later in the book). Consequently, the concept was tested in the wrong context and subsequently abandoned by most of the organizations that attempted to execute it. Rather, SLM is—and must be—organizationally pervasive to yield full benefit and achieve its full potential. Therefore, from the start, it should be noted that SLM is not about marketing. Although marketing may be one component, it is not the driving function or force in its application.

This time around, however, there seems to be a heightened understanding of the concept and a more compelling reason for incorporating its function into the operating milieu of the organization, and savvy organizations are doing just that. If the prevailing environment is not enough to motivate organizations to consider the concept of SLM, one driving force might prompt hospitals and health systems to implement the model: competition.

EMERGING COMPETITION

Although several other factors explain why SLM is a fitting organizational configuration and why every hospital and health system should seriously consider its application, the one that will likely prompt healthcare executives to move is the emergence of new competitors in the field. With everything else to consider, healthcare administrators must now face this daunting threat. Competitors range from specialty hospitals that carve out the high margin services such as cardiology or orthopedics to physician-owned diagnostic centers.

Physician Centers

Many factors contribute to the rise and prominence of these emerging physician centers as competitors. On the physician side, declining real incomes as well as lackluster returns from the equity markets are prompting physicians to consider owning centers that offer not only increased convenience and control but also the prospect of financial benefit. While the conditions that prompt doctors to enter into such arrangements can certainly be appreciated, these arrangements present an increasing dilemma for hospital executives who face eroding margins and increasing costs. To lose the higher-margin services such as cardiology, as well as the diagnostic elements, is not only problematic but can threaten the very economic viability of the hospital.

Dependency on Core Lines

For example, for those hospitals that provide cardiology, it is usually the number one service line in terms of contribution margin, often representing between 25 and 50 (and in some cases higher) percent of the hospital's total margin. To negatively affect a core service line is to erode the financial stability of a hospital. The same can be said, but perhaps at a reduced level, for other services or procedures, whether it be orthopedics or diagnostic imaging.

While SLM is not the silver bullet to resolve the threat of emerging competition, the organizational structure can improve the hospital's or health system's ability to either preempt competition, compete effectively against such competition, or pursue a middle ground of partnership with potential competitors in the market. In basic terms, SLM provides the focus on the core services or areas that are most important to the hospital, assigning distinct and direct accountability to an individual or individuals to monitor the dynamics of the market and ensure that the organization is optimally positioned to protect, defend, and expand in those areas that are mission critical.

Too many organizations have made the near-fatal error of assuming that the behemoth size of hospitals or systems acts as a market shield against the encroachment of a smaller, less-substantive niche player. However, experience has proven that such thinking is fundamentally flawed as specialty hospitals have entered markets with firmly established larger competitors and have readily and rapidly taken control of the market. The issue at stake in these markets is often the very thing that makes SLM such an attractive and relevant model: The ability to target the key stakeholders (patients and physicians) as well as establish a clear identity with the community and consumers. Community or tertiary hospitals may be known for many things, but a "heart hospital" is immediately positioned as having the expertise in that area.

Traditional Competitors and Limited Capital

An effective and well-organized SLM structure establishes the organizational architecture, so to speak, to both anticipate the needs of the market and the movement of potential competitors. The default strategy of waiting until the competition is at the gates is almost always detrimental and sometimes seriously deleterious to an organization's perceptual position and financial results. More will be said on the specifics of competing against emerging competitors in subsequent chapters. Suffice to say at this point that SLM is, by its very nature, the most appropriate organizational configuration to confront and compete with this very real threat.

Along the same lines, SLM can be a very effective mechanism in dealing with more traditional competition. And even though the industry is facing the prospect of increased volumes from the aging population and heightened utilization caused by less-restrictive health plan administration, competition will always play a major role in healthcare.

VALUE IN THE CONCEPT OF CO-OPETITION

SLM can be not only one of the best models for assessing competition, allocating resources, and designing strategy, it can also provide the framework for "co-opetition," the idea of collaborating with competitors. This has proven highly successful and financially beneficial for many organizations. They have found that collaboration is often better received and more highly rewarded and/or reimbursed than the more traditional route of competing for services. Because surveys have shown that many people believe the competitive nature of healthcare has led to unnecessary duplication of equipment and services, collaboration is usually well-received in the community. And, as studies have repeatedly shown, collaboration—while difficult, time consuming, and politically charged—does have economic benefits (Palmquist, Coddington, and Fischer 2000).

The current environment in healthcare is such that executives need to rethink the time-tested approaches and historical modes of operation. With the demographics and the nature of health insurance (with less-restrictive health plans) mentioned above, the industry faces a future of what the Health Care Advisory Board terms "profitless growth." Unlike the good old days when hospitals would count every patient as economically beneficial because of the contribution to overhead and fixed costs, the capacity constraints that currently confront executives and that will continue to do so are forcing administrators to rethink their approach to services.

The increasing number of patients accessing care through emergency rooms and relying on emergency departments as their "medical home" is resulting in a heightened ratio of medical cases to surgical procedures and, as expected, the diminution of higher-volume cases. This unfavorable mix will only increase as the number of the uninsured rises and access to primary care physicians diminishes. Consequently, each organization must review its patient mix and its service line structure frequently and consistently to determine if the portfolio of services it is offering can financially sustain the organization over time and through more challenging periods. Failure to do so will result in situations like those so many hospitals found themselves facing in the late 1990s—the kind that requires eleventh-hour assistance or dramatic turnaround expertise as a result of the organizations' poor economic performance and dire financial straits.

FRAMEWORK FOR ALLOCATING CAPITAL AND RESOURCES

Once again, SLM provides an elegant and sophisticated structure for measuring and monitoring results as well as allocating operation and capital resources. Of singular interest in this area is the allocation of capital resources. Over the next five to ten years, capital availability will loom as one of the most significant challenges healthcare executives must confront. As the population ages and demand for care increases, capacity constraints will be one of the chief concerns keeping CEOs and other operators awake at night. Given the recent downturn in the equity markets, investment income has dwindled considerably, placing greater tension on operating income statements as well as balance sheets. Hospitals and health systems—especially not-for-profit organizations—are reluctant to spend too much on capital expansions or go to the bond markets too frequently for fear of losing their favored status in bond ratings.

Consequently, capital allocation is critical now and will remain so in the foreseeable future. A solid service line structure is one of the best evaluative mechanisms for determining where to allocate capital and, perhaps even more important, where *not* to allocate capital.

Capital allocation is one of the most compelling reasons for ensuring accurate and objective portfolio analysis. Relative ranking and capital budget discipline is integral to good SLM configuration.

SUMMARY

This book is designed to outline the "rules" for service line success. These rules, while not necessarily rudimentary, are also not rocket science. Chapter 2 outlines each rule in sequential order, with each subsequent chapter detailing the specifics around how to put these practices into place. The rules are an outgrowth of my experience with SLM over the past 17 years in the healthcare field. They are broad guidelines designed to help healthcare managers better understand the conceptual reasoning behind the service line structure and to incorporate that model into the organization.

REFERENCES

Health Care Advisory Board. 2003. *Financing the Future: State of the Union 2003.* Washington, DC: Health Care Advisory Board.

Palmquist, L. E., D. C. Coddington, and E. A. Fischer. 2000. "It Doesn't Come Easy. A Survey of Hospital CEOs Gives Insight into Collaboration." *Health Forum Journal* 43 (3): 34–7, 50.

CHAPTER 2

Eight Essential Rules for Service Line Success

THIS CHAPTER OUTLINES and briefly describes the eight essential rules necessary to establish an effective service line program and achieve service line success. Each rule is given a synoptic description at the outset of the chapter. The chapter also provides the rationale for the chronology and methodology and serves as a summary overview of the entire SL orientation.

THE ESSENTIAL (AND SEQUENTIAL) RULES

As elementary as it may sound, there are basically eight rules to service line excellence. If an organization follows these rules (or steps), it is likely to experience favorable results in a relatively short time frame and position itself better within the market and against its competitors. The eight rules are as follows:

1. Define the lines
2. Measure what matters
3. Narrow down to two or three
4. Create the optimal organizational design

5. Assess market position by service line
6. Develop appropriate business plans
7. Compete aggressively and strategically
8. Apply the model throughout the organization

These rules are not only essential, they are also sequential. They should be accomplished in chronological order to maximize the effectiveness of the service line management (SLM) model. Failure to do so will result in a suboptimal introduction and execution of SLM. The inherent elegance of the SLM model will come into clear focus as the organization progresses through these eight rules.

One of the big challenges of service line orientation (and consequently its reason for failure in so many organizations) is that there is too much to understand and implement at the outset. The value of following these eight rules is that they rapidly get the organization to the point of core business identification and survival-crucial services and operations.

Herein lies the beauty of the model. In a relatively short time, managers are able to identify and isolate those services that contribute the bulk of the revenues to the institution and the major segment of the operating margin. Following is a summary of each of the eight rules and why it matters in sequence and relevance.

Rule 1: Define the Lines

This seemingly fundamental and rather rudimentary step is where many organizations struggle the most. It is also the "make it or break it" rule because it sets the stage for how the process will proceed and how likely the model will succeed. Think of this rule as the foundation of a home or building. If the foundation is hastily designed and poorly constructed, the entire edifice will likely be substandard.

Defining the lines is difficult work because this is where politics, traditions, and territory enter into the process. Yet the organization's leaders must steel themselves for the task and take an objective and industry-comparable approach to ensure that the subsequent rules can be realized. This rule is probably where the most time will be spent and the greatest discussion will occur. It may also prove the most frustrating, as there will be a sense that the momentum is slowing and the model is doomed. As one very wise individual once noted, "Start right and you will end right." The converse is true: Start wrong and you will likely end wrong.

In application, this definition of service lines needs to be nothing more than a decision by senior management on how the lines will be defined. As will be shown in Chapter 3, DRGs or ICD-9 codes can be used for the inpatient and ambulatory payment classifications (APCs) for the outpatient measure (if applicable). These are not the only criteria that can be used. For example, some organizations have determined that ICD-9 codes provide a more in-depth picture for the inpatient segment of the line. Criteria based on clinical alignment or medical staff organization are not recommended because they are difficult (if not impossible) to measure against market competitors or national benchmarks.

Rule 2: Measure What Matters

Once the criteria have been established for determining how the service lines will be defined, the next rule is to establish which measure matters most for the key stakeholders of the organization. This should not be a difficult exercise, and it may prove illuminating to actually quantify the measure by service line.

By measures or metrics, I am referring to those measurable statistics or quantifiable components that determine the success or failure of the organization. These are the items that get reported to the board of directors, the community leaders, senior management, or whatever group is responsible for evaluating the ongoing success of the hospital or health system. Obviously, some *financial indicator* should be included in this group, perhaps even two or three financial indicators. The key is to have something that can be measured for each service line, such as net revenue, operating income, or contribution margin. In some cases (e.g., investor-owned facilities) the economic metric might be EBDITA (earnings before depreciation, interest, taxes, and amortization). This is the gauge that matters most to for-profit firms in the aggregate, so why not take it down to the service line level?

Some kind of *volume measure* should also be used, such as total discharges for an inpatient consideration or number of tests or surgeries for the outpatient component of the service line. The volume metric might also include a relative gauge such as market share or market growth for that particular service line. The ability to measure service line position against competitors is one of the main reasons for selecting definition criteria (Rule 1) that are quantifiable and transferable across facilities and throughout the industry.

Other metrics that might be considered in this second rule include a *quality indicator*, such as complications or mortality indices. As with market share gauges, depending on the data source the hospital or health system uses, these can be measured relative to area competitors or peer group hospitals within the industry. These gauges of quality are becoming increasingly more relevant as regional employer coalitions or national assemblies, such as The Leapfrog Group, become more involved in the operational component of the industry.

Rule 3: Narrow Down to Two or Three

Once the metrics have been determined to gauge service line success based on overall organizational criteria, the next rule is to narrow the service lines, or the areas of focus, down to two or three core lines. The core lines can be singled out by using the metrics identified in Rule 2 (measure what matters) using a series of analytical matrices and a variety of data-dependent graphs and tools (a few of which will be depicted in Chapter 4, which deals with this subject in greater depth).

The culling of service lines is a crucial step for three reasons. First, it makes the implementation of SLM much easier to accomplish. Too many organizations begin the service line process and organization with 9, 13, or even 18 lines. One hospital had identified 23 service lines. When asked which were priorities, the CEO said, "all of them." Although there is nothing inherently wrong with having several service lines (although 23 is definitely too inclusive), the key is to zero in on those lines that can make or break the organization.

The second reason for focusing on two or three lines is management attention and resource commitment. If the organization identifies ten lines that are going to demand management time and attention, the entire effort will be diffused. Therefore, it is far better to identify just two or three that can realistically be monitored and managed at the highest level as well as at the crucial mid-range level where the core accountability will likely reside.

This latter point leads to the third and final reason. By narrowing the focused field down to two or three lines, upper management can take the time and expend the resources to staff those lines with dedicated people. This has proven to be far more productive and effective than piling one more added responsibility on an already overworked middle manager or administrative-level executive. Adding on responsibility is much more likely to occur if the organization has identified ten or so service lines, thus making it nearly impossible to pursue a course of hiring an outside manager for each service line or elevating an existing one if that is determined the better thing to do. Additionally, as will be discussed in Chapter 5 (organizational structure), the notion of organizing a matrix team for each line has produced very favorable results for many hospitals. However, that likely will not occur if the hospital or health system has upwards of ten lines at the outset.

This step is actually what has made many successful companies in other industries what they are today. They have learned to apply the *Pareto Principle*, or the 80:20 rule, which states that 80 percent of an organization's successful performance (however it is measured) is derived from 20 percent of its products or services. The healthcare industry would be well served to better understand and more artfully apply this time-tested principle of management.

Rule 4: Create the Optimal Organizational Design

Once the number of lines has been narrowed to those two or three on which the hospital or health system is highly dependent for its ongoing success, the organizational structure can be established. As noted above, narrowing the field down to a small number of crucial lines makes expending the time and effort to find the right individuals and the proper organizational complement for the high-priority service lines much easier.

Many variables for assigning service line responsibilities must be considered (and these will be explored in greater depth in Chapter 6), but one of the most important is the internal-versus-external candidates decision. Ultimately, attitude and personality matter more than inside-versus-outside considerations. Some internal candidates with an entrepreneurial flare have made excellent service line managers. Organizational dynamics and stakeholder considerations are other important issues. For example, in a heavily specialist-dependent line, an established clinical manager who enjoys a stellar reputation and outstanding rapport with the doctors may be the logical candidate. On the other hand, local market dynamics may call for someone who brings fresh perspective and creative approaches to a line that has been stagnant for a time and needs rejuvenation.

The other critical element of organizational constitution is the support group that backs up the dedicated manager or director of the service line. This can be a task force (not usually recommended), a matrix team (highly recommended), or a hybrid of the two. Whatever the design, each line should have a cadre of individuals representing a wide array of critical functions that provide input and insight into the operational component of the service line. The options, with their pros and cons, will be explored in greater detail in Chapter 6.

Rule 5: Assess Market Position by Service Line

Once the organizational design is determined and the individuals who have been given responsibility and accountability for managing and building the lines are in place, a competitive assessment is the next step to take. At first, this rule may seem similar to Rule 3 (narrow down to two or three), but that rule involves only an internal analysis. This segment of SLM concentrates on assessing the two or three core service lines against the chosen comparative organizations or benchmarks. Those benchmarks may be peer groups (similar size and services throughout the state or country) or local and/or regional competition.

The metrics used to make the competitive assessment would definitely include those identified in Rule 2 (measure what matters), but it could also involve additional measures that might be relevant to that particular line and the specific market dynamic. For example, the competitive assessment would likely include several qualitative measures (such as public surveys to measure awareness and quality perception) as well as many measures that include a more broad-range assessment by several of the key stakeholder groups—especially physicians. Several of these measures (and how to derive them) will be discussed in Chapter 7, which provides more information on this facet of SLM.

The competitive assessment is important for a number of obvious reasons, not the least of which is capital allocation. In these times of constrained capacity and restricted capital many hospitals must make tough decisions. One of the most daunting decisions deals with which expansion or development opportunities are best suited for the long-range success of the hospital or health system. This type of decision should never be made without a thorough understanding of how individual services are positioned—perceptually and strategically—against competitors. Importantly, that list should include existing, as well as potential, competitors.

In Chapter 7, the discussion of niche player, specialty hospitals, and physician ventures comes into play the most. As noted earlier, one of the best arguments for developing or strengthening the service line structure is to counter or preempt these new competitors, which threaten to erode the economic core of many larger hospitals and health systems in the country.

Rule 6: Develop Appropriate Business Plans

Once the competitive assessment is completed, the organization can develop the business plan for each service line. Actually, some organizations may decide to include the competitive assessment as the introductory element of the business plan in the environmental analysis section. That decision is entirely up to management and depends on how business and strategic plans have been developed within the organization in the past.

The healthcare industry tends to spend so much time on the environmental assessment (market analysis, or whatever it might be termed) that the market backdrop becomes the main focus of the planning effort. By the time audiences have heard all the data and statistics, they are so worn out and worn down with data that they want to speed through the objectives and strategies. That is reverse logic and suboptimal business planning.

The objectives should demand the greatest amount of time and devotion, for that is what will drive the organization's resource allocation and ultimately determine whether it has met its reason for being. Unfortunately, these objectives are often derived in haste or frustration, rather than deliberated at length and revisited for reasonability. More will be said on this in Chapter 8, but executives must recognize that objectives determine strategy and strategy drives the organization, or at least it should.

Strategies are those carefully worded statements of action that should be well planned as well as thoughtfully and deliberately executed. Each major strategy should come under scrutiny. It should help achieve the associated objective and thereby enrich the overall organization. Metaphorically speaking, if too much time is spent on the frame of the picture (the environmental analysis), few individuals will have the patience or the endurance to concentrate on the brushstrokes of the painting.

The business plan needs to eventually get down and dirty with the details. These are best left in the appendix, or somehow kept in the background. Such details are likely to be bland and granular, and consequently they do not need the attention (or even perusal) of key audiences like the board or senior management. Nonetheless, having them in writing is good for review and accountability.

Rule 7: Compete Aggressively and Strategically

One difference between this approach to SLM and the previous one is that this time less emphasis is placed on the actual execution segment. As noted earlier, the first wave of service/product line management became so focused on promotion and marketing—the execution elements—that these elements overshadowed the organizational aspect. Consequently, this generation of SLM has only one rule and one section for the execution segment.

Focusing on one rule and one section is by no means meant to diminish the importance or the significance of execution. Rather, this new approach emphasizes the need to put the organizational building blocks of definition, design, and distillation into clear focus. In other words, if those aspects are done and done well, then the execution phase will have a higher probability of achieving the overall objective, which is to position the organization in a more competitive way.

Many organizations will struggle in this area. Not only does this require successful design and execution of the messaging component, it also requires differentiating the service line vis a vis the competition. This involves strategy, pure and simple—although in this field strategy is not that simple. Our industry is undergoing significant change, and thus the ability to gauge the key components and market variables is increasingly more difficult.

Rule 8: Apply the Model Throughout the Organization

Once the organization has piloted the concept of SLM with one or two service lines and proven that it is viable and invaluable, then more service lines can be identified, more managers assigned, and more matrix teams (or multifunction groups) appointed.

Applying the model throughout the organization is an important next step and final rule for two key reasons. First, it conveys to everyone in the entire organization that they will have their day in the sun and that this is not an initiative or strategy meant only for the high-profile, high-margin elite. Second, it will help make the notion of SLM pervasive throughout the entire organization and better ensure its continuity over the long term.

The ultimate success of this rule depends on the necessity that it sequentially follows the other rules and especially pivots off of Rule 3 (narrow down to two or three). By piloting and proving the concept with two or three service lines, the organization is in a much better and more probable position to extend the concept of service line structure throughout the entire organization, or at least over several more service lines. The organization that wants to implement the model in its entirety, at least at the outset, actually is more likely to abandon the concept before it can be proven viable. However, given the nascent (and arguably foreign) nature of SLM in healthcare, incremental implementation and execution provide a much more likely road to success.

SUMMARY

These eight rules, if incorporated and followed, should establish a model and a framework for SLM in any hospital or health system. The subsequent chapters describe in greater detail each of the rules. As mentioned at the start of this chapter, the rules are best understood and applied in the order listed. If understood and implemented in a way that is applicable to the local market, these rules should assist hospitals and healthcare systems in focusing on the lines of their business that matter most, while at the same time meeting the demands of a volatile and unforgiving market.

CHAPTER 3

Rule 1:
Define the Lines

THIS CHAPTER FOCUSES on the need to clearly define how service lines will be determined. This definition is critical in the overall development and planning for service lines, as it will be the basis by which the service lines will be prioritized, evaluated, and assessed. The chapter describes several options for defining the service lines based on data configurations and offers the most reasonable and workable approach to defining service lines.

DEFINITION IS FUNDAMENTAL

The first rule of service line success is that lines need definition. Unfortunately, defining what constitutes a service line is one area where most hospitals and health systems get bogged down. This fundamental definition is what often confounds many managers as they attempt to place parameters on the nature of service lines within the organization. As elementary as it may sound, much of the initial momentum is often lost in the area of definition.

For example, if a hospital determines that it will define its service lines based on project-oriented or event-specific criteria, it may determine that the new MRI should qualify as a service line. Or perhaps the fact that the implementation of bariatric surgery at the hospital merits added attention and marks it as a candidate for service line status, or status is conferred by the recruitment of a well-known surgeon in a particular subspecialty such as pediatric oncology. This type of structural definition poses many problems. First, this approach lacks comparative data sources by which to measure market success. Without measurable data within the organization to provide relative value of that particular segment, the managers will not perform the critical task of prioritization. This must be done to ensure that limited capital is being allocated to those areas (service lines) where it will have the greatest return. The organization's resources must be parceled out based on the overriding strategy for the organization, which is based on the relative strength—both financial and operational—of each area.

SLM is fundamentally an objective tool for prioritizing the core areas that will ensure the long-term success of the organization. Such prioritization and subsequent allocation cannot occur when the gauges for determining service lines do not allow comparison of data, both within the organization and throughout the market.

WHAT SERVICE LINES ARE NOT

Given that service line definition is sticky and tricky, it may be useful to delineate what does *not* constitute a service line.

- A department or function that does not produce revenue that is reimbursed by commercial or government payers (e.g., the gift shop) would not be considered a service line.
- A service that is actually a subset of a service line (e.g., pediatric oncology; the service line is oncology and pediatric can be broken out) does not constitute its own service line.
- An umbrella category that is too loosely defined to be able to measure (e.g., medical services) is not a service line. The service line may be general medicine, but "medical services" could involve several lines such as medical cardiology, medical oncology, and so forth.

- Services that may be in vogue but are difficult to track and to measure (e.g., alternative and complementary medicine) should not be designated as service lines. For most systems and in most areas, such services lack the benchmark data necessary for comparison as well as traditional and established reimbursement sources. This could be set up in a separate category, but in the early stages of SLM development it would only confuse matters.

Some people will review this list and dismiss it out of hand if they have established service lines that fall into one or several of these areas. If this strategy is working and the organization has done an effective job of prioritizing the many possible service segments down to three or four (which will be discussed in Chapter 4), then by all means continue. What usually happens, however, is that an organization's executives first determine what service lines they want to offer, and then they designate those service segments or department functions as service lines. This approach lacks the crucial first step of arraying all the relevant and contributing components or areas of an organization's business and then objectively determining which areas are of greatest value to that organization. That value determination can be based on criteria ranging from financial to mission fulfillment, but it should be based on relative measures of strength and long-term success as well as objective data that can be reassessed over time. Without such a value determination it becomes nearly impossible to effectively prioritize or to objectively and strategically allocate management time and organizational resources.

DEFINE BY DATA AVAILABILITY

A good SLM strategy should serve as the means to both streamline strategy as well as to focus resources; otherwise the structure is suboptimal. The only way to ensure that it serves this purpose is through the use of sound and reliable data. Thus, the first determination should be the criteria for identifying the service lines.

Although it is certainly not the only way, using a diagnosis related group (DRG)–based data configuration and evaluation for the inpatient definition of lines is recommended. The reason for using DRGs, at least at the outset, is the availability and comparability of data within markets and across service lines. This was not always the case. When service lines were first being developed in the mid- to late 1980s, data were not all that plentiful. However, a few firms exist now that can readily provide detailed and sophisticated data analysis for 1 to 30 service lines. Of course the latter number is unwieldy, but a prominent firm (Solucient) does produce data for over 18 service lines.

Starting with that many lines—12 to 18—is not necessarily a poor beginning. In fact, at the outset, the more service lines that can be compared using the same data elements the better. The beginning of the project is the ideal time to identify several lines and ensure that all are in the evaluation pool. The time to narrow them down—culling the lines—is after the first phase.

The significant challenge for some service lines comes into play with diagnoses and procedures (or causes for admission) that seem to cross clinical guidelines. For example, oncology is one of the most challenging, if not *the* most challenging, line to define. A few options exist. One, and perhaps the easiest and most workable, is to use the definition outlined by national data firms (i.e., Solucient) and apply the same classification of DRGs as they do. Another option is to do what was done in the early days of product management—apply the criteria of "majority rules," which means the appropriate service line for each DRG is determined by the percentage of cases based on the primary diagnosis. For example, if a particular DRG had 51 percent cancer-related diagnoses, then all of the admissions for that DRG accrued to the oncology product line. This may not seem terribly accurate or even necessarily representative, but sometimes such a definitive decision is needed to move the organization beyond "analysis paralysis."

Other categorizations or data-defining options that can be considered for the oncology service line (and for other lines where applicable) include the following:

- *ICD-9 codes for all the major diagnostic categories (MDC) designations.* These codes (e.g., MDC 1, diseases and disorders of the nervous system, through MDC 25, human immunodeficiency virus infections) can be used for all the admissions, irrespective of primary/secondary diagnosis or subsequent admission status. A designation of ICD-9 coding allows the hospital to more accurately reflect what is actually occurring within the oncology line, something that is admittedly lost by using only a DRG designation.
- *ICD-9 designation based on primary and secondary diagnosis for the admission.* The advantage of using just the primary/secondary diagnosis is that it may more accurately reflect the admissions/patients listed in the oncology service line vis a vis other service lines or disease classifications where, upon admission, the patient was also determined to have a cancer-related diagnosis or illness.
- *ICD-9 designation for only the primary diagnosis.* This is the same rationale as above (for primary and secondary diagnosis), but it narrows the definition and classification to an even greater extent.

These are some of the options that can be used in determining how best to define/classify the oncology service line. The challenge with using this type of classification for oncology (and other relevant lines) is that the ICD-9 classification is not as easily compared to regional and national benchmark data. For this reason, many hospitals and health systems opt to use the DRG basis. Although this may not accurately capture oncology volume, at least it produces a framework where the data are comparable to those of other hospitals (competitors), allowing for financial analysis.

One other option employed by some hospitals and health systems is to maintain two definition methods, or keeping two sets of books. The first set of classification/definition is the DRG method, which can be used to aggregate the entire hospital and draw market comparisons across the region or country. The second classification is just for those service lines (e.g., oncology) that require more drilling down to the ICD-9 or APC level to more accurately represent and depict what is actually occurring within those more complex and multidisciplinary lines. This second set of classifications can be delineated in the business plan, with a footnote or appendix addendum that clearly explains and differentiates between the two data descriptions and definitions.

While this may seem like more detail than the reader ever wanted to absorb, the truth is that not many diagnoses (or DRGs) fall into the gray area, or outside of the oncology service line. Most of the diagnoses are fairly clear-cut, and the assignment to the appropriate service line will not be difficult. The key thing, which cannot be stressed enough, is to move past the hand wringing and head scratching over how to classify and get to the stage of organization-wide analysis. The detailed definition and category assignments can always be modified as the data collection improves and the actual execution of strategy takes shape.

USE THE DATA SOURCES AVAILABLE

Once the definitions have been solidified—in essence clarifying which DRGs constitute the identified service lines—then the data can be gathered on each line. Many organizations have the capacity to conduct this analysis with their existing resources or via the services of outside data-management firms with which they already contract. Interestingly, many senior leaders are not aware of the data resources to which they already have access or the kind of reports that can be generated. A first step in determining what is required to assemble and then array the data would be to survey the information systems, financial, and perhaps planning staff to get a sense of what is available through existing resources such as the cost accounting system, purchased data management, or even system-wide reports. For example, the HCA organization has its own database that closely parallels that of Solucient's service line classification. Therefore, for HCA hospitals, the data are already in place to effectively establish and monitor service lines.

The value of defining the service lines based on data configuration will be demonstrated throughout the subsequent chapters in this book. Many of the hospitals and health systems that might currently consider their organizations in the service line mode have not effectively defined their lines. However, as will be shown in later chapters, there are great advantages to doing so—primarily the ability to gauge the performance of the lines against local, regional, and national competition. Another advantage lies in the very essence of healthcare delivery, which is the reimbursement structure.

DRILL DOWN ON THE DATA

Because DRGs are the operative classification for getting reimbursed from the government for inpatient procedures (through Medicare and Medicaid), a data-defined service line enables the service line manager and the team or group responsible for the service line to analyze the financial appropriateness of each individual DRG as well as the service line in its entirety.

For example, when service lines were first being defined back in the late 1980s at Sacred Heart Hospital in Eugene, Oregon, defining financial appropriateness became one of the primary roles of the service line team. Once the line had been defined, the plan had been outlined, and the basics were in place, the service line team evaluated each DRG within the defined service line for oncology to determine if the reimbursement coming from the government was sufficient to cover the costs to provide the service and to meet the financial targets of the hospital.

Once that kind of analysis is conducted, the SLM team or manager can begin to develop and implement strategies on an individual DRG basis or ambulatory payment classification basis for outpatient services. This kind of drill-down by procedural code or category is much more readily accomplished when the service lines are defined by data classifications—just one of several good reasons for defining the lines based on data divisions.

Once the "audit" of data resources and service line classification has been conducted, the next step is to assign responsibility for the development and analysis of the data, based on the service lines identified and the classifications determined.

LINE UP THE LINES

The process of arraying the lines is an instructive and illuminating one. Relevant data for the identified service lines should first be assembled, then verified, and then arrayed. Although the data can be arrayed in several ways, the best methods are those that involve easily understandable and compelling graphics. A portfolio grid or analysis is an excellent way to display a vast amount of data along two (or perhaps three) evaluative criteria. For example, Figure 3.1 takes several service lines and presents the data using three variables. The y-axis is the measure of contribution margin per discharge—a good financial gauge and one that is relevant to every hospital and health system. The x-axis measures average annual growth for that particular service line. Something like a growth measure can either be based on historical data or projections. Either way, the growth coefficient gives a sense of the service line's potential.

Figure 3.1 also displays a third measurement variable—the relative total contribution margin for each service line, which is represented by the size of the "bubble." This measure gives management a sense of the financial "weight" of each service line.

Figure 3.1. Service Line Analysis

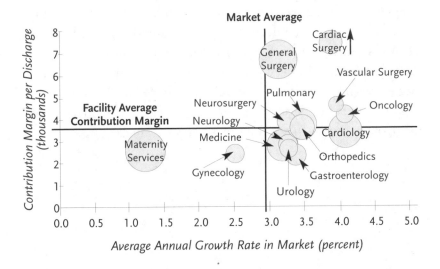

Note: Size of bubble represents total contribution margin.

A line may have stellar financial performance but may exist in a climate of stagnant growth potential. This would argue for a strategy of protecting current volumes, but it may not provide sufficient rationale for investing sizeable resources or capital commitment in that particular service, because the growth potential is limited. Conversely, a service line may have the potential for significant growth but may not offer the promise of high margin. This situation (less-than-sustainable margin) can either be the service line's foregone fate, or it may be a matter of more accurately coding the procedures. It could also be a function of the reimbursement not keeping up with the resources required to deliver the service. In the case where reimbursement has not kept pace with the resources required to provide the services or deliver the care, a case may be made for lobbying the payers to reimburse more in line with the costs of the procedure and the organizational resources required to render the service.

SUMMARY

Defining the lines is a fundamental first step in establishing an effective service line strategy. Far too many hospitals do not take the time or make the effort to effectively and consistently define their service lines. Such a lack of clearly defined lines will likely result in loosely defined objectives, nebulous evaluation metrics, and slippery accountability assignments. Without clearly defined lines, an organization will fail to develop properly the service line model and will likely never realize SLM's full organizational value.

CHAPTER 4

Rule 2:
Measure What Matters

THIS CHAPTER OUTLINES the metrics, or criteria, that each organization should consider for both prioritizing the identified service lines and measuring their success relative to the competition and against the goals/objectives that will be established in the business plans for each line. These determined metrics are very important to establish at the outset. They will provide the baseline against which the success or failure of the service lines will be judged as well as the basis for assessing the performance of those assigned to and accountable for each service line.

DEFINE THE METRICS THAT EQUATE TO SUCCESS

One of the key components that is frequently missing in the design and development of service lines is the early establishment of the metrics for gauging success. All too often these are identified well down the implementation path as an afterthought and, as such, are far less likely to be representative of and consistent with the organization's overall and long-range strategy. Consequently, what sometimes occurs is a disjointed or even out-of-sync evaluation and assessment of service line performance relative to the rest of the organization. For example, one service line manager was evaluated on his ability to attract new patients to a line, with little consideration for the operating margin of the service line. Therefore, he was successful in increasing overall volume, but in disease classifications that were either lower margin or no margin. The outgrowth of this situation was that the operating margin for the line diminished and the resources and attention allocated to this service line siphoned off resources from higher margin lines, to the detriment of the organization's financial picture. Yet the manager was only doing what was expected of him.

Quantitative Metrics

This anecdote illustrates the acute need for the organization to identify early and distinctly those metrics that represent the key areas of emphasis and focus on which accomplishments will ensure the long-term viability of the organization. These measures—and there need be only five or six—must become the basis for prioritizing the service lines, establishing achievable objectives, and then ultimately evaluating the success of the strategies adopted in the business plans for each line (as described in later chapters). However, if the leadership team has first identified the metrics that matter most, the exercise will prove invaluable when the time comes to develop the business plan and its critical components such as defined organizational goals.

For many organizations—especially during these times—the salient metrics will likely be financial in nature. These would include measures such as net revenue, operating margin, or total contribution margin. Consideration may also be given to cash on hand or some other measure of liquidity as well as other balance sheet criteria that influence an organization's bond rating. As organizations are pressed to expand capacity to meet the increasing demands of an aging population, access to the capital markets (which for many hospitals is through the bond markets) will become increasingly more critical.

In developing the list of key metrics that matter most, senior leadership merely needs to pose the question, "What do we discuss the most at our executive leadership sessions and at board meetings?" For most organizations, the answer to that question will be "financial statements" or "economic measures." That is not always the case, but experience teaches that much of the discussion these days involves financial results.

Within that category of financial measurements, however, the item that matters most will likely vary by the market and the type of organization. For example, at the investor-owned or for-profit hospitals the statistic that gets the most attention is EBDITA, or earnings before depreciation, interest, taxes, and amortization. This is sometimes rearranged to be EBITDA—the order most often used outside healthcare—but the calculation remains the same. EBDITA is the driving factor for organizations like HCA, Tenet, and other for-profit chains. This is what budgets are based on and what plans are oriented toward.

In the not-for-profit world, the calculation that matters most is likely to be *operating income* or *net margin*, depending on how the organization or system refers to its bottom line. (In the not-for-profit world, the term "profit" is not used much, so it is replaced by "margin.") Some organizations like to consider the gauge of contribution margin (what's left over after variable costs have been considered) to assess the ability to contribute toward fixed costs. A few organizations will focus on *net revenues* as a critical gauge, although concerted emphasis on revenue is becoming less relevant as executives begin to recognize that not all volume is beneficial (i.e., profitable) and that margin considerations are increasingly more germane. Few organizations even give serious consideration to the artificial top line of *gross revenue*, as it has virtually no value or relevance except perhaps as a shadowboxing exercise to show what the organization *should* have received for the provision of its services. But few individuals or audiences (including the media) care to hear that story or frame of reference anymore.

Quality Metrics

Some organizations may focus on *quality measures*, such as complication or mortality indices, as these may be driving factors for positioning the organization. Significantly, such quality measures are becoming a crucial metric for influence-wielding and even volume-steering bodies such as business coalitions or industry groups (e.g., The Leapfrog Group). This may intensify over time as employers exhibit more interest and wield more clout. One thing to consider in long-range planning as it relates to quality metrics is the likely configuration under a single-payer system or a centralized decision-making authority (i.e., nationalized medicine).

Having quality measures as part of the key metrics is a sound strategy for several reasons. First, it sends a message to all stakeholder groups that the organization is serious about quality and committed to monitoring it, comparing it, and enhancing it. Second, a concerted focus on quality measures is likely to have the desired effect of improving clinical outcomes. In management science, this dynamic is often referred to as the "Hawthorne Effect." The name is derived from an employee study (at a GE plant in Chicago from 1927 to 1932) that basically holds that those behaviors or indicators that are frequently monitored and measured will usually show improved results. Finally, given the increased emphasis and scrutiny on quality outcomes, organizations that place their quality metrics on display are getting the jump on organizations like The Leapfrog Group and state data agencies and, to a certain extent, seizing control of the information that is reported and reviewed by the public.

For these reasons and many more, organizations should include at least one quality metric in the basic five or six criteria by which the service lines will be identified, arrayed, and prioritized. The truth is that these metrics may not ever become public knowledge, but if they do (and some organizations may even choose to make them public), then having a quality metric or two will resonate well with any audience.

COMMUNITY NEED

Another area that should be considered among the five or six fundamental metrics by which the organization prioritizes its core service lines is community need. This could also be referred to as mission fulfillment, although community need is more readily understood outside healthcare circles. Community need is somewhat like the quality measures in that it is qualitative and also will carry greater public acceptance.

A few examples of metrics that could be included under community need would be

1. A certain level of care for the uninsured
2. Educational efforts centered around health challenges and issues
3. Response to specific predominant unmet needs

The Uninsured

The issue or challenge of the uninsured is receiving more attention and awareness than ever before. People are starting to realize that the high number of uninsured is a dilemma that affects everyone— directly or indirectly, financially as well as socially. Although some may realize that hospitals bear the brunt of the problem, very few understand to what extent hospitals deal with this rising and perplexing dilemma. Some states have a minimum level (usually expressed as a percentage) of charity care that must be provided to meet tax-exemption stipulations.

Yet most people, even in those states where such regulations are in effect, are not aware of these stipulations. A hospital or health system that establishes a metric for the level or dollar value of charity care provided, and then makes that metric public, is educating the community about an important function of the hospital. Such forthright and candid disclosures may also serve to buffer criticism and concern when hospitals are placed in the spotlight as the cause for increasing prices (something that is occurring to a greater extent). Because most Americans have no clue as to how healthcare finance functions, information on funding of the uninsured provides a valuable framework for dialog and a backdrop for discussing other financially related issues within the industry.

Education

Healthcare institutions can be invaluable vehicles for communication about local health-related issues. Some hospitals set goals in terms of communicating to their communities the effects of serious illnesses that are lifestyle related, such as obesity, diabetes, certain cancers, and heart disease. As the hub of healthcare, hospitals and health systems lend both credence and clout to messages about health issues. They are also arguably in the best position to coordinate such messaging in concert with health associations (e.g., the American Heart Association, American Diabetes Association, and American Lung Association), community groups, employers, and other interested parties.

Some hospitals and health systems have education departments, so incorporating educational campaigns and initiatives into the mix by measuring the level of awareness, participation, or another metric is quite natural. As with the uninsured issue, health and fitness concerns are beginning to surface, commanding more media attention and public concern. The rising problem of obesity has been targeted by some health advisors and experts as a greater health concern than smoking. Hospitals or health systems that take the initiative and lead the charge in an educational and assistance campaign on obesity will not only glean a great deal of favorable publicity, they will also be performing a valuable service to the community.

Unmet Needs

Many health systems focus on those areas of the business that will provide a meaningful and sustainable return on their investment. Although this is natural and in most cases appropriate, areas of unmet needs (e.g., teenage pregnancy, childhood immunizations, and a host of disease-related support groups) within the community should also be considered. While addressing these needs will not likely (or at least not in the foreseeable future) provide a financial return, it speaks to the mantra of "improve the overall health of the community" encompassed in most healthcare organizations' mission statements.

By establishing a metric that deals with such unmet needs, the hospital or health system is basically saying that profit is not everything and that meeting the needs of the community is also very important. Some skeptics may scoff at this type of reasoning, but healthcare leaders must recognize the perceptual box they may be placing themselves in. The growing perception (similar to that in the early 1990s) is that hospitals and health systems are too focused on making a profit. Even though most of us in the industry know that the average (bottom line) margin is less than 3 percent for hospitals across the country, the public either does not know that fact or does not believe it.

Consequently, including metrics like "prominent unmet need" helps to diffuse the misperception of "profit before patients" and helps instill in the public's mind the notion that hospitals really are about caring, not just cash. And, more importantly, as with the other two metrics discussed above, it brings the organizations back to their reason for being, which fundamentally is to ensure and enhance the healthcare of the residents of the community.

SELECTING SIX SALIENT CRITERIA

Based on the broad categories discussed here, an organization can choose the five or six measures with the most significance to the key constituencies or stakeholder groups charged with monitoring results and ensuring viability. These measures or metrics can be arrayed in a number of fashions, but using some form of dual-axis matrix is recommended (see sample matrix in Figure 4.1) as it provides a graphic snapshot and an easy-to-understand visual for experts as well as novices (such as community residents, should the organization choose to make its metrics public).

For example, the six salient criteria (or metrics) for prioritizing the service lines might look like the following for a not-for-profit, community-based hospital:

1. Net operating margin (for the entire service line)
2. Combination of growth and market share relative to competition in the area
3. Percentile ranking for complications vis a vis national averages
4. Percentile ranking for mortality vis a vis national averages
5. Total dollars of charity care provided for that service line
6. Opportunities to fulfill unmet community needs within that service line

Once the data for these metrics have been gathered for all the service lines, it can then be arrayed for each measurement, and the core lines identified. For the quantitative measures, the critical lines—such as cardiology, orthopedics, or surgery-based lines—will stand out rather readily. The other criteria are not so easily predictable, which is one reason they make for an interesting part of the mix.

Importantly, the criteria can be assigned different levels of "weight." For example, net operating margin may be assigned a ranking weight of 40 percent for that one measurement, which may actually be low by some standards based on the relative weight financial metrics are given. The growth and market share metric may be

Figure 4.1. Key Metrics: Value to Stakeholder Group

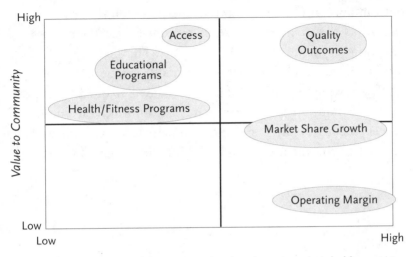

Value to Financial Supporters (i.e., bond market, shareholders, etc.)

assigned a weight of 20 percent, giving the other measures a relative ranking weight of 10 percent each.

The ranking mechanism or formula used will depend on the goals, philosophy, and strategic direction and orientation of the organization. By diversifying the measures a bit so that not only financial and volume measures are included, the organization sends an important message that success means more than merely meeting or exceeding the bottom line. Such a message emphasizes that hospitals are in the business of caring and not just focused on caring about the business.

SUMMARY

Whatever measures are selected and weights assigned, early identification of what matters most will assist all those held accountable for the success of the service lines. Additionally, the metric identification, followed by the core service line selection, will help the organization focus its resources on those critical areas essential for long-term viability. By identifying the measurements or metrics most important to the organization, senior leadership enables and empowers the management team to concentrate their time and attention on the things that matter most. This delivery of focus is invaluable, especially in times of flux and frustration.

By knowing the handful of metrics that will frequently be measured and monitored, the management team can better filter and process the myriad messages and countless distractions that would otherwise deter their focus and inhibit their success.

CHAPTER 5

Rule 3: Narrow Down to Two or Three

THIS CHAPTER DESCRIBES how an organization can identify and focus on the two or three service lines that are absolutely essential to its long-term success. It also discusses how the organization can begin to consider streamlining its overall portfolio by reducing, consolidating, or eliminating underperforming service lines.

IDENTIFYING THE CORE SERVICE LINES

Once the service lines are arrayed and prioritized based on the metrics established in Chapter 4, the organization then selects the two or three lines that are essential to its long-term success. Although not necessarily easy (expect some degree of organizational angst), this paring down is essential. This is where the SLM model first proves its value—facilitating the discipline to concentrate on the two or three service lines vital to the future of the organization.

The concept of core service lines or areas of business is nothing new to the industry and may not be all that new to healthcare organizations. However, the SLM approach uses objective data and sound strategic reasoning in selecting the best of all the hospital's many areas of operation. Consequently, the criteria for prioritizing the key service lines should be indicative of the organization's culture as well as representative of the key stakeholder groups.

PRIORITIZING THE LINES

The prioritization that takes place with the SLM model is nothing more than a data-driven implementation of the 80:20 rule, or what is correctly known as the *Pareto Principle*. Vilfredo Pareto was an Italian economist whose research in the early 1900s has been advanced since its first economic use and applied to modern management theory. The 80:20 rule maintains that 20 percent of an organization's (or individual's) effort produces 80 percent of its key outcomes, such as revenue, margin, or profitability. The secret to successfully instituting and executing Pareto analysis is to correctly identify that 20 (or so) percent and then be willing to concentrate the organization's planning and resources on those high-producing areas.

In the previous chapter we discussed how the organization must outline and clarify those metrics that define its success. These metrics include the standard measurements of organizational effectiveness and long-term viability such as operating margin and market growth. These two variables, along with the others, can be displayed graphically to effectively demonstrate the relative strength of the service lines within the organizations.

Figure 5.1 demonstrates such a representation for one particular hospital. This graph, referred to as a "portfolio analysis," depicts all of the hospital's service lines in what is sometimes called a bubble chart. This portfolio analysis can then become the basis for selecting the two or three service lines that will receive most of the organization's time, effort, and resources (i.e., capital expenditures, upgraded equipment, and marketing dollars). As can be seen in Figure 5.1, this hospital should ensure that cardiovascular surgery and cardiology receive the bulk of the organization's resources and

Figure 5.1. Service Line Analysis

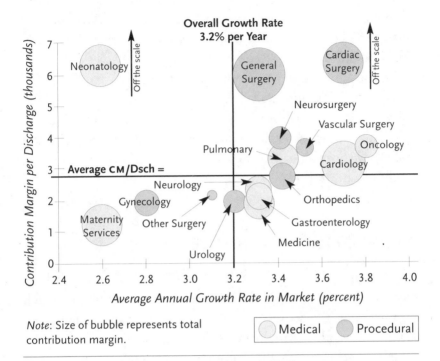

Note: Size of bubble represents total contribution margin.

attention. Conversely, based on the information displayed, this organization would not want to devote too much time, energy, or resources to women's services, as that is a line that is neither growing nor very profitable.

As basic or elementary as this kind of analysis may seem, in many healthcare organizations, the leading service lines—those that are absolutely critical to the hospital or health system's success—do *not* receive the kind of attention that is commensurate with their contribution to the overall success of the enterprise. In fact, because they have proven so successful over time, there is a counterproductive tendency to regard them as "givens," and thus the organization concentrates on areas that represent future revenue streams or margin centers.

Although this counterproductive strategy is a precarious one to follow, it has been played out in many markets. Hospitals have not committed the time and resources to high-margin areas such as cardiology, and they realized too late their mistake, as specialty hospital, niche players, or physician-led initiatives drained off their business and eroded their revenue streams and margins. This does not mean, however, that a commensurate match between the service line and the focus it receives will necessarily stave off competitive forces or automatically create market barriers to entry. What it does mean in many cases, however, is that if more attention had been paid to key physicians and core services, the organization might have been able to create its own center, alleviating the need for physicians to find "outside" partners.

PROTECTING THE CORE

Based on the testimony of both the physicians who partner with specialty organizations and the executives who work for such organizations, the doctors who consider outside arrangements do so for reasons other than financial. The arrangement often provides benefits that the hospital has not delivered, such as convenience of surgery times, nursing expertise, or some other advantage. Whether hospital executives want to believe it or not (and some will always remain skeptical of this), most such arrangements were not initiated solely (or perhaps even primarily) based on economic considerations).

Whatever the case, a good prioritization of core service lines should lead the organization to concentrate its time, attention, and resources to ensure that critical lines of business remain viable and robust. This means that the organization recognizes the absolute imperative to protect and defend core areas as well as commit the resources necessary to grow those segments of the business. The realization and commitment usually begin with the clear understanding of just how much those areas affect the organization, and perhaps a "what-if" exercise to assess what it would mean should the organization lose a sizeable portion of any or all of those critical lines.

SUBDIVIDING THE SERVICE LINES— MEDICAL AND SURGICAL

In many cases, such as the one depicted in Figure 5.1, hospitals or health systems choose to subdivide the surgical component of a service from the medical component, such as cardiovascular surgery from cardiology. This type of separation is recommended. Separating the medical component of a service line from the surgical gives a much more definitive picture of how the overall service is performing. Such segmentation also provides the institution with the ability to identify the significance of the financial contribution of the procedural and the medical areas within the same discipline. For most facilities, the surgical or procedural segment of the specialty will provide higher margins, and considerably higher in many cases.

Consequently, hospitals are feeling a capacity crunch, but the increased volume of patients is producing a deteriorating, and potentially unsustainable, financial dynamic as the procedural cases are gravitating to specialty hospitals or physician-owned centers or hospitals. Therefore, dividing the medical segment from the surgical provides the organization with both the necessary data to assess the relative contribution (margin and otherwise) of the subsegments as well as the capacity to monitor the effect over time.

Referring back to Figure 5.1, the same is true of the neonatology service line split out of women's services. Admittedly, many hospitals do not have NICU capabilities, but the concept of carve out is instructive. Figure 5.1 demonstrates that the women's services line is, in and of itself, in the lower-left quadrant. That line is one of this organization's poorest financial performers and could theoretically be considered a candidate for scaling back or "demarketing." However, in the case of this organization, such a strategy might prove to be short sighted and economically unsound as it could have the undesired effect of reducing neonatal cases, one of the organization's highest margin contributors.

This information is shown more transparently in Figure 5.2, which depicts the total contribution of each service line or sub-

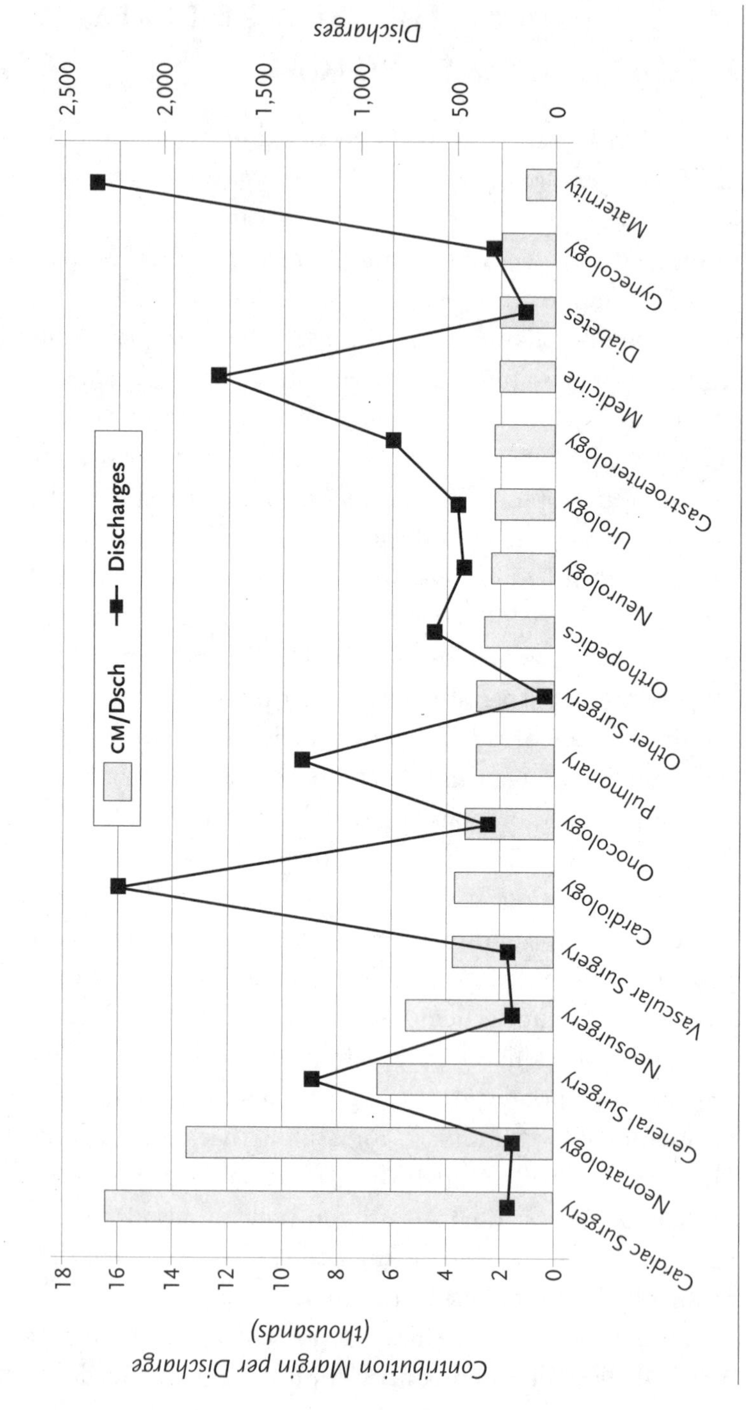

Figure 5.2. Contribution Margin per Discharge, by Service Line

component of the service line. As can be seen from this graphic, neonatology represents the best financial performer for this organization—even higher than cardiac surgery. Again, the value of dividing the surgical from the medical, or the subspecialty from the overall service line, is to highlight those areas that, even though part of a larger service line, are vitally important to the economic well-being of the hospital.

Different Slices of Service Line Performance

These graphs also depict an important managerial exercise, which is to take several different "snapshots" of the organization to depict the data several ways; this is especially important for an organization that wants to consider several different variables in determining its core service lines. Case in point, the criteria that have been presented in the previous graphs are primarily financial, with some consideration for market growth. Yet obviously several other relevant, and for some organizations perhaps even more essential, criteria must be considered. These could include ensuring access, providing services, accomplishing the mission, and aligning with physician interests. Some of these determinants are more readily quantified than others and thus more easily graphed. Those variables that are more qualitative in nature can be assigned numerical values based on consensus of key stakeholders or stakeholder groups or the assessment of senior management.

Whatever technique is employed, the fact remains that most if not all criteria for assigning and ranking organizational value can be, and should be, quantified and depicted in a readily visual fashion. An example of a more "qualitative" grid is shown in Figure 5.3, in which the two determinants are "mission critical" and "stakeholder sensitive." These two subjective criteria are assessed using "high" and "low" as the evaluative determination, which serves to provide a different perspective on two variables that can factor quite heavily in an organization's ongoing strategies.

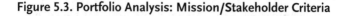

Figure 5.3. Portfolio Analysis: Mission/Stakeholder Criteria

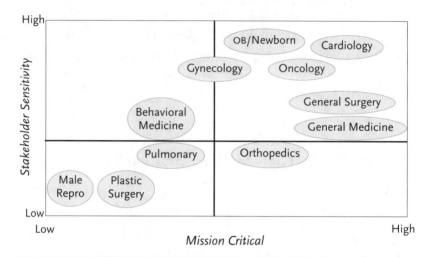

In truth, for most organizations in these times, organizations will likely use criteria that are financially oriented, market-growth/market-share based or a combination of the two. However, that does not preclude any organization from also factoring in criteria of mission fulfillment or community need. These criteria will likely prove to be highly important—especially for not-for-profit governance bodies (such as the board of trustees). These types of criteria should also be considered in light of other key stakeholder groups such as community leaders, donors, politicians, and even the media.

At the very least, qualitative analysis that factors in variables other than economic and market share will demonstrate to several groups that the organization considers many essential variables in assessing which lines matter most. This analysis will also prove valuable (as will be shown later in the book) when the organization considers which service lines should be consolidated, shifted to another provider or delivery source, or eliminated altogether. In that kind of analysis, the organization's aims are quite different, as it considers why a line should be given time and resources (or even why it exists) rather than focus on the lines that matter most. By initially factoring in these other evaluation criteria for the key service lines, the organization will have become familiar and comfortable with the exercise so that it will be an integral component of service line analysis.

SUMMARY

One of the most important things every organization can do in these times of limited capital and unlimited need is identify the areas of operation that matter most. The service line structure offers the framework to objectively identify the two or three service lines that, in reality, constitute the essence of the organization and account for the lion's share of its financial stability.

By using the criteria for evaluation discussed in earlier chapters, senior management can graphically highlight those two or three service lines that offer the best potential for growth as well as the highest contribution to the bottom line. These are likely to be the driving criteria for selection of the core service lines, but the organization can also factor in qualitative considerations such as community benefit, mission fulfillment, or perceived stakeholder value.

Whatever the criteria chosen for paring down the service lines to a manageable two or three, this exercise enables management to concentrate its resources and attention on critical services. In many cases, these services represent the leading source of financial stability. In an era of niche competitors, health systems are likely to be vulnerable to competitive market forces ranging from physician ventures to specialty hospitals. A focused service line effort is one of the best, if not *the* best, structures for shoring up the organization's base as well as fending off the competition.

CHAPTER 6

Rule 4: Create the Optimal Organizational Design

THIS CHAPTER DISCUSSES options for organizational design for the core service lines identified. Although no clear-cut definitions of the optimal organization exist, choosing certain constructs offers clear advantages. The chapter also probes some considerations relative to job description and characteristics for effective service line managers.

MANAGERIAL STRUCTURE

Once the two or three essential service lines have been identified and selected, a managerial structure must be established to ensure success for each of the core services. Although many options can provide varying degrees of success, certain key components should be incorporated into an organization's design. Sufficient authority and adequate accountability must be inherent within the management design.

To that end, two options—both proven successful—should be considered for managing service lines. Although both are quite divergent in terms of orientation, they have common elements and metrics that could also be applied in other structures. These fundamental tenets ensure the effectiveness of the model, perhaps more than the model itself does.

OPTION 1: MATRIX DESIGN WITH DEDICATED SERVICE LINE MANAGER

When the concept of service line management (SLM) was introduced and implemented in the mid-1980s, one of the most popular models for organizational design was a matrix configuration. In a matrix design, the manager is not given direct-line responsibility but rather has to manage individuals and functions that are essentially "dotted line" reports. This structure was adopted from organizations like Procter & Gamble, where the concept had been tested and proven over decades. The value of the matrix model is that it spreads the responsibility across several functions and departments and thus encourages both input and ownership throughout the organization. This was particularly germane and valuable in the early days of product line/service line management, when the nascent concept needed broad-scale awareness as well as pervasive acceptance. To that end, the matrix design still has value and applicability and should be considered as a viable means of implementation. This is especially true in organizations unfamiliar with service line structure.

Downside of Matrix Design

The downside of a matrix orientation is twofold. First, the nature of healthcare administration or medical management tends to be rather traditional and thus hierarchical. Healthcare administration follows the military model, which is as close to the antithesis of matrix management as a management style can get. Consequently, many healthcare executives may be uncomfortable with matrix management. It requires not only a new mindset but also a different reporting and accountability structure. Some senior managers in healthcare say, "I want to have one person ultimately responsible." That dynamic is still possible under a matrix design, but the input measurement and feedback cycles are different than those under the traditional structure.

Second, the matrix organization is not as "clean" in terms of single-point responsibility or accountability. Interestingly, the inherent value of the matrix orientation—spreading ownership and encouraging cooperation throughout the organization—can also be one of its biggest deterrents because it also spreads the accountability. Some executives are uncomfortable with that concept. However, the matrix (or team approach) has been proven highly effective not only in consumer goods organizations but also in leading managerial models. The concept of team product launch or product management is one of the core ideas to emerge from the Deming approach (the total quality improvement movement of the 1980s based on data gathering and monitoring, which is credited to management guru W. Edward Deming). This approach is often cited as a driver of improved quality and "owned" responsibility.

Natural Fit for Healthcare

In healthcare circles the matrix design is both natural and fitting, as the very nature of the delivery model is multifaceted. An individual entering a hospital interacts with a variety of functions that crosses department boundaries and requires considerable coordination. It is completely natural, therefore, that a business planning and strategy execution team or group would be effective in optimizing the success of a service. Realistically, the individuals involved in the matrix team that supports an SLM approach would become involved with the line at some point in time and at some degree. It would follow that involving them at the outset and throughout the process

would only improve their contribution and enhance their ownership in the success of that particular line.

The Value of a Dedicated Service Line Manager

The core member, the leader of the matrix team, is the service line
(SL) manager. The SL manager is already critical to any organization
design, so this is an element that does not change materially, irrespective of the ultimate management structure. However, under a
matrix organization a little more consideration may be given to the
scope of the role and thus to the individual who fills it. Based on
experience, a dedicated SL manager is the optimal approach for any
configuration. If the organization can institute an organizational
structure of dedicated SL managers, it is likely to experience greater
success.

Dedicated managers are more prone to success for two easily
understandable reasons. First, and somewhat obvious, is the fact that
the SL manager is able to concentrate his or her complete attention
on the service line. Senior managers, department directors, or assis-
tant administrators who assume the responsibility for a particular
service line along with their other duties will almost always be grav-
itationally pulled to their existing or former responsibilities. A manager with a single focus is more likely to succeed than someone who
is being asked to multitask and cross function.

The second reason for a dedicated manager's success has more
to do with the organizational dynamic and perception than the individual's focus or ability. A strong message is sent and relative value
assigned to that service line and the overall concept of SLM when it
has a dedicated manager. If the responsibility for a service line—even
if it has a high profile and a good margin—is given to a current manager as an add-on, the cachet given to the concept and to the line
will be less than if a devoted SL manager is given the same responsibility. There is clout in focus and greater empowerment in dedicated responsibility.

The Service Line Manager's Role in Assembling the Team

Admittedly, not all organizations can afford (or think they can afford) dedicated service line managers. Considering the inherent value of the Pareto analysis, however, if an organization carefully and thoughtfully defines and outlines the intrinsic organizational value of its three or four service lines, executives quickly recognize that devoting one individual (even if highly compensated) to a cardiac line is a small investment to ensure large revenue retention. The first few steps of arraying the lines and highlighting the impact or significance of the top three make it easier to allocate resources to those critical service areas.

Once the SL manager is assigned or hired, he or she can be instrumental in identifying the remaining members of the matrix team. No standard selection criteria exist, but the list below identifies some of the functions that should be considered for the team:

- Finance
- Marketing or public relations
- Clinical leadership (perhaps the department director)
- Nursing (unless the clinical director fills that role)
- Lab
- Medical advisor (physician in that specialty area)
- Ancillary functions (where applicable)
- Diagnostics area
- Coding or billing (if the financial member does not represent those functions)
- Senior management or administration (vice president or equivalent)
- Materials management
- Other functions highly involved in the identified SL function

This is by no means a comprehensive list, but it is representative of the type of individuals and the functions that should be on the team and it will add value and contribution to the success of the service line.

OPTION 2: CLINICAL DESIGN WITH ADJUNCT COMMITTEE STRUCTURE

The second option for service line design involves the use of a clinical manager who is already in a supervisory role for that particular area but who assumes the expanded responsibility for the development and strategic direction of the line. This usually encompasses an expanded definition of the manager's job description and broader accountability for the financial success of the entire line, not just the more narrowly defined clinical evaluation. For example, this structure might involve taking the nursing director over obstetrics and making him or her the SL manager for all of women's services. In this instance, the director must assume much greater responsibility with a more broadly defined area of control.

Pros and Cons of Clinical Design

This design is probably easier to implement than the matrix design, as it follows more closely the traditional hospital orientation and organization. Most hospitals already have department head structure established, so this design involves working within that framework while augmenting the existing structure to incorporate the input and involvement of other functions.

In this organizational design it is absolutely essential to incorporate other functions—such as marketing, finance, planning, and facilities development—within the service line planning and implementation design. If the organizational design is based on the traditional structure of clinical orientation, the supporting services and departments are not as likely to be included or at least not given the same degree of involvement and clout. Some organizations think (somehow) that by just adding the moniker of SLM they will favorably affect the outcome.

To be successful, a shift must occur in the organizational design and thus the market orientation of the new structure. This requires a design that still incorporates the authority and accountability mentioned at the outset of this chapter, and it must extend to the key functions within the hospital or health system.

MANAGING SERVICE LINES WITHIN A MULTIHOSPITAL SYSTEM

This question is often asked, "What is the best configuration for managing service lines within a health system that has several facilities?" The answer is quite dependent on the model and the strategic orientation of the system. If the system is pursuing a clinical center-of-excellence approach—where it is focusing its efforts and resources on one flagship facility or campus—then it is probably best to centralize the SLM responsibilities at the system level.

If, on the other hand, the system is intent on developing the service lines at each facility, with little in common among those lines (perhaps other than marketing and contracting), then it is likely best to have service line responsibility at each of the facilities. There are several reasons for this approach.

First, to reiterate the inherent value of the concept, service line orientation is designed to get close to the customer and to anticipate the needs of the market. This is difficult to do on a regional or multisystem level as healthcare is local. Having one service line manager for multiple facilities (and often in diverse markets) diminishes the ability to engage the key customers (especially physicians). This would be especially relevant in markets where physicians are considering pursuing entrepreneurial ventures or joint operating agreements with specialty players. Consequently, the ability to anticipate the needs of the market and to preempt the emerging power players would be almost nonexistent.

The second reason for a decentralized structure lies in the nature of the organization. As emphasized throughout this chapter, there is great value in getting the input and involvement of many contributors within the facility framework. This is difficult to do at the system level, as things tend to be so general and theoretical to be considered or rendered trite. It is better to operate and analyze at the level where the customers are interacting—within the facility. People do not usually relate to cardiology services across a system; they relate to how cardiac care is delivered at a particular hospital with a specific doctor and an individualized team of caregivers.

SUMMARY

This chapter has presented the two most commonly applied design structures: A matrix organization with a dedicated service line manager and a clinical design that incorporates more of the existing (and traditional) hospital orientation with expanded responsibility but still with direct reporting relationships. While each option has its benefits and deterrents, the dedicated service line manager working within a matrix design more closely parallels the model that has been tried, tested, and proven in other industries, and even within many healthcare settings.

The organizational design component for a SLM structure is an important decision. It should not be considered lightly nor viewed as something that can be simply overlaid onto a current operating structure with existing employees. Considerable thought should be given to which managerial design best suits the needs of the market and the goals of the organization. Obviously every organization is different, and therefore what works for one hospital or health system may not work well for another. However, a multifunctional service line team working in a matrix model with a dedicated service line manager as the leader of the team, is the preferred model. By its very nature, this model seems to more easily synthesize the inherent benefits of SLM, and optimize the resources of the organization.

CHAPTER 7

Rule 5: Assess Market Position
by Service Line

THIS CHAPTER OUTLINES several strategies for competing effectively within the market on a service line level. A particular focus is on competing against niche players or the new competition from physicians currently on staff at the hospital. The chapter suggests why niche players have an inherent advantage and discusses options, from collaboration to outright competition, in dealing with such.

THE NEW COMPETITORS

One of the greatest advantages of a well-organized and well-executed service line design is its ability to position the organization effectively against competition. This is especially relevant in these times when the stiffest competition is likely to come from a new crop of market players. Over the next five to ten years, hospitals and health systems may be more preoccupied (and rightfully so) with the competitive threats they face from specialty hospitals, physician ventures, and single-service providers. These "focused factories," as Regina Herzlinger (1999) calls them, represent a clear and present danger (or at least a substantive threat to existing healthcare providers) for the following reasons:

- They are singularly focused on one specialty or service line.
- They often have physician financial support and operational input.
- They can more easily be identified and positioned in the minds of patients.
- They are often more aggressive and savvy at marketing.
- They do not have the same degree of "social responsibility" in treating a broad economic cross-section of patients.
- They are more maneuverable in a changing market.
- They often operate more efficiently.

This is just a partial list of the differential advantages that specialty players bring to the equation. Larger hospitals and health systems have believed that their strength (and inherently superior model) lies in their depth and breadth. However, consumers (or patients) and physicians have basically said in many markets, "who cares about the girth of an organization—we're fundamentally interested in the extent to which you are meeting our needs." The sense of imbedded market advantage, which health systems once naively assumed would accrue to their benefit, has been eroded by the success of these new competitors.

Consequently, the response to such competitors must be certain, unflinching, and pronounced. Too many hospitals or health systems have waffled in their competitive response or sent mixed signals to the doctors and the public about their position. This leaves the window of opportunity wide open for new entrants to establish their position and achieve an early advantage with consumers.

Case Study in the Southwest

One example is worth citing. A rapidly growing and highly attractive market in the Southwest was home to two large health systems. One was an entrenched religious system that had a solid reputation and the leading market position. The other was an investor-owned system that had been formed during the merger era of the mid-1990s and was gradually gaining share on the not-for-profit system. Both systems had strong cardiac programs that accounted for a disproportionate share of revenue and margin.

Given the dynamics of the market—two strong systems, heavy managed care, younger-than-average population, and more-than-one strong cardiology group—the setting did not look all that favorable for a specialty cardiac hospital to thrive. Despite this seemingly saturated market, MedCath Corporation (headquartered in North Carolina) opened a cardiac facility. Within two years the facility had assumed the number one position in the market in terms of consumer awareness (as measured by market research) and taken about a third of the volume away from the larger, more entrenched systems in the area.

In essence, the MedCath facility was able to come into an established market and create a perception among the public that it was the very best place to go for anything related to the heart, from diagnostic testing to heart surgery, because its singular (or main) medical focus was the heart. MedCath was able to accomplish this by having a name—Heart Hospital—that definitively communicated what it did; by assembling and engaging a large number of cardiologists and cardiovascular surgeons as investors; and through heavy marketing that broadcasted its existence and its singular expertise. By capturing the public's attention and awareness, it was also in a better position to negotiate with managed care companies and to work with employers on services ranging from executive physicals to cardiac rehabilitation. MedCath's smaller yet more concentrated hospital provided some valuable lessons summarized below for all organizations facing similar market dynamics:

- Take all competition seriously, especially entities that threaten the core business.
- Never underestimate a new market entrant because of its size or experience.
- Never presume what the market wants or how the consumer will respond.

- Strike preemptively, not reactively—the first to market will usually remain first.

SERVICE LINE STRUCTURE HELPS THWART COMPETITION

A service line structure actually provides one of the best, if not *the* best, operating and organizational structures to anticipate specialized competition. If a service line structure is in place with managers assigned to the core lines, the managers and their service line teams should be the first to know about any potential competitive threats. Part of a service line manager's job, as well as the team's, should be to keep abreast of market dynamics. Doing so requires constant contact with the key stakeholders related to the service line. This would obviously include physicians—both those loyal to the facility as well as those loyal to the competition.

One reason that established hospitals and health systems have taken such a pronounced hit from the specialty players is that they have not had dedicated individuals or teams assigned to monitor the market. Consequently, in many instances, by the time they get word of a physician uprising, a competitive inroad, or a major defection, it is too late—the damage is a fait accompli for that market. Attempts to salvage the situation are too often stop-gap or reactive. All one has to do to validate this premise is to look at what has happened in many of the markets where new competitors have entered. The responses have been anything but calculated and the subsequent success far from stellar, as evidenced in markets such as Indianapolis, Austin, Oklahoma City, or Sioux Falls where niche players have entered the market and captured consumer awareness and market share.

The Need for Well-planned and Preemptive Strategy

The best time to develop strategy is early in the process when several variables are still in play and multiple options are available.

When strategy is planned at the eleventh hour, with very few options, the execution is usually short sighted, overly expensive, and predictably reactive. As with so many things, timing may not be everything, but it is critical. One of the greatest benefits of SLM is that, if it is well organized, high profile, and ultimately accountable, it buys time because it incorporates the discipline of business planning and ongoing market reconnaissance. Such market assessment ensures more predictive than reactive strategy.

This notion that highly effective, dedicated service line managers will earn their salaries several times over just by focusing on existing and potential market dynamics and competitive activity is something that healthcare leaders have been either remiss or unable to grasp. Unfortunately, too many senior executives mistakenly believe that this type of reconnaissance is the purview of marketing directors or department managers. Granted, some organizations do have individuals in these roles who consider it part of their responsibility to keep their finger on the pulse. Although these individuals may achieve admirable success, there is always the dilution and distraction factor for an individual whose role is either broad (i.e., marketing director) or operationally in-depth (i.e., department director). Whatever the reason or the distraction, the fact remains that the traditional hospital organizational structure is not well suited for anticipating competitive threats or for successfully countering such threats once they become a reality in the market.

SERVICE LINE MANAGERS AND THE ROLE OF MARKET INTELLIGENCE

An organization that has a functioning service line structure should position itself to take advantage of its more conducive orientation. Service line managers should provide regular reports on competitor initiatives, marketing thrusts, and forays, either formally through business plan updates or informally through periodic review. This structured system for reporting gives senior management a more accurate picture of what is occurring in the market as well as what to anticipate. This type of reconnaissance and review also gives senior executives invaluable guidance and framework for their strategic planning and capital-allocation decisions. Without it, the consequence is often reactive strategy (which is really not good strategy at all) or suboptimal execution done in haste and without proper lead time, market research, and stakeholder input.

Many of the pitfalls of faulty initiatives and flawed strategy could be avoided if a process and structure existed for periodic reports from the field. Very few organizations, however, institute a competitive assessment update. Surprisingly many organizations, including some of the larger and more financially viable for-profit organizations, do not even have a formalized strategic planning process. This begs the question, "If the large for-profit companies and their hospitals do not have structured and rigorous planning as part of their regimen, why should organizations bother?" The answer can be found in the roller-coaster history of investor-owned and not-for-profit hospitals and health systems.

Look at most of the well-known firms, whether not-for-profit or for-profit, and a disturbing trend of peak-and-valley financial performance becomes evident. Although this can be expected given the nature of the industry and the unpredictability of the variables that affect healthcare, the counter argument is that an industry with such volatility should strive for even greater efforts at planning. The benefits of tracking the competition and anticipating competitive strategy is one of the more compelling reasons for pronounced and pervasive SLM orientation.

MANAGING THE COMPETITION

Good service line managers will become as familiar with the competition as they are with their own organization. In the consumer goods industry, product or brand managers spend a great deal of time studying the moves and motives of their key competitors, keeping tabs on what they are doing from both an operational and a marketing sense. Doing so helps a manager not only to anticipate the effect on the market but also prepare to respond in a way that will effectively neutralize the competition's efforts.

In healthcare, this often takes on the look or feel of "me-too" initiatives. Healthcare has earned a reputation for being an industry of lemmings that follow the competitor across the street or the seemingly successful hospital across the country. This type of reaction is often just that—a reaction that is not grounded in thoughtful process or carefully planned execution. The value of a service line orientation when competing—especially against smaller and more nimble players—is that it subdivides the organization into units that *can* more effectively compete because they are given the authority and the accountability to track competitor movement and then to respond (not react) accordingly. These unit managers keep senior management informed on both the competitor movement and the recommended strategy to counter and contend with the competition. In essence, a service line structure makes managers more acutely aware that they are not only responsible for their own line but for the competitor's as well, because what the competition does will have a direct impact on their business. This concept of "managing the competition" is not very prevalent in the hospital field, but it is in other industries, and it will pay valuable dividends for those organizations that understand and practice it. As the old movie line goes, "I keep my friends close, and my enemies closer."

Opportunities for Co-opetition

Not that competitors are enemies, nor should they be regarded as such. In fact, one of the outcomes of monitoring actions by competitors may be to offer a strategy involving collaboration. The concept of *co-opetition*—cooperating or collaborating while still competing—is beginning to take greater hold in this industry. For example, the idea of time-share operating rooms, a concept tested by Tenet and other organizations, is an excellent example of innovative co-opetition.

The model has worked very well in other industries, especially in the high-tech sector. For example, the design and development of SemaTech as an industrywide organization to help the American technical companies compete against their foreign counterparts is regarded as a very successful model. SemaTech was formed in the early years of high-tech emergence as a way for U.S. tech companies to share best practices and establish industrywide synergy to more effectively compete against foreign tech firms. It was financed by the larger firms and viewed as a kind of nonpartisan enterprise to aid all the U.S. firms.

Correspondingly, there may be opportunities for competing hospitals or health systems to find common ground, mutual interest, and economic benefit in pursuing collaborative ventures. Studies have shown that collaborative ventures between competitors, while difficult to design and execute, prove to have good financial results. Careful tracking of competitor movement may provide advance notice of possible beneficial collaborative arrangements.

Joint Ventures with Physicians

An example of co-opetition is the possibility of joint ventures with members of the medical staff. As physicians experience declining practice incomes and greater demands on their time, they want to gain more control over their lives and their economic future. Consequently, many are splintering off and developing enterprises that directly compete with the hospitals or health systems that for decades have provided them a venue to practice their profession.

Some healthcare executives view this as a kind of treason or at the very least a competitive threat. Savvy executives, however, will anticipate the interests and needs of key members of their medical staff and begin evaluating opportunities for partnership with the doctors on ventures that are mutually beneficial and legally permissible.

These types of ventures offer all parties the option to collaborate rather than compete outright, and although the ultimate outcome may not be as economically attractive for the hospital or health system, it may prove better than losing a large share of business to the competing physician ventures.

The hospital or health system that frequently and faithfully monitors and manages the competition will find that its overall strategy will likely improve as the organization undertakes a more structured and calculated approach to assess and analyze the strategy of its competition. In many industries competitor analysis is fundamental, whereas in healthcare it is too often limited to the annual or tri-annual (or however often the planning process occurs) review of the market as part of the environmental assessment. However, if such assessment and analysis occurs only on an infrequent and limited basis, the significant moves of competitors (either existing or potential) will not be detected in a timely fashion.

As with so many components of service line structure, the service line manager and his or her colleagues bring great value to the organization in terms of both the information they provide and the business planning discipline they exhibit. If the service line structure is adequately and accurately functioning, the competitive response—ranging from aggressive competition to possible collaboration—will be more readily identified and more easily achieved.

SUMMARY

The notion of competition in the American healthcare system is as entrenched as it is productive. Service line orientation offers an excellent framework for assessing an organization's competitive position and then determining the optimal strategy. In an era of emerging competitors who offer single-service emphasis—known as "niche competitors"—a service line strategy can help transform a larger, inflexible, and lethargic organization into a responsive and focused entity that can compete more effectively.

A dedicated service line manager, supported by a multidisciplinary team, can more readily anticipate market needs and more successfully preempt or respond to competitive threats. One such response platform may be co-opetition, where the hospital or health system chooses to partner with a specialty player or enterprising physicians. Whatever the selected mechanism or model for competitive response, a service line structure is an excellent organizational framework for matching the resources of the organization to the needs and demands of the market.

REFERENCE

Herzlinger, R. E. 1999. *Market-Driven Health Care: Who Wins, Who Loses in the Transformation of America's Largest Service Industry.* New York: Perseus Publishing.

CHAPTER 8

Rule 6: Develop Appropriate Business Plans

THIS CHAPTER FIRST establishes the need for annual business plans for each service line identified as part of the core. The chapter further describes the components of those business plans, providing a framework as well as a template for business plans that will outline the basic components for success within the SLM model.

ANNUAL BUSINESS PLANS

Once the organizational structure and framework has been established and the individuals selected and assigned to fulfill the roles, the next rule to understand is that few business units or lines will succeed without a detailed plan. Therefore, key to service line success is the development of a well-researched, well-organized annual business plan. This is a critical step that is sometimes overlooked or given short shrift. However, one of the great values of the SLM model is the emphasis on sound and structured planning.

The notion of business planning is where the SLM construct presents one of its great differentiating values. Creating a business plan for each service line offers the organization the ability and opportunity to break down the strategic plan into manageable units with tactical plans. In far too many organizations, the literal breakdown between plan and execution occurs because there is no mechanism or structure to "operationalize" the plan at the practical and measurable level. Good SLM planning should alleviate that disconnect and obviate that dysfunction.

Business Plan Provides Direction, Accountability

The business plan that is developed at the service line level performs a dual role. If done correctly and thoughtfully, it provides input and direction for the strategic plan and, more importantly, becomes an actionable document derived from the overarching and broader strategic plan. In essence, it creates a symbiosis between the strategic plan and the business plans—an interdependency that should make both documents more substantial and relevant.

For that reason the business plan cycle for service lines should be in sync with the strategic plan. At the outset, the strategic plan for the organization should precede the service line plans and thus be the root document and driver for the plans. To that end, the service line plans should not deter or detract from the strategic plan. If the service line plans do not support the overall strategic direction and goals of the organization, the organization may be forced to decide which has more relevance—the service line plan or the strategic plan—and determine which requires and receives the limited resources. Service line plan diversions from the strategic plan are not all that uncommon. Such diversions create a situation where the broad-scale goals of the organization may not be satisfied, despite considerable success within the service line. Certain hospitals and health systems (not a few), have had stellar individual programs or service lines but have struggled as an organization.

Strategic Plan and Business Plan Linkage

The lesson then for senior executives is to have a strategic plan to serve as a guide to provide broad course direction and operational parameters, such as financial targets and available resources. The service line plans then become a contributing component or a complementary offshoot of the umbrella strategy. While this might seem rudimentary, having no strategic plan at all is even more common than having diversions from the strategic plan.

Organizations faced with the need to isolate one or two key areas, such as cardiology, often launch with a business plan for the service line without a more encompassing document (i.e., strategic plan) to provide the necessary framework. The danger with this approach is that parameters are never established and a sense of relative efficacy and weighted contribution is never achieved. So when the service line team, for example, suggests (through its detailed business plan) that what the line really needs is a new center of excellence to provide differentiation from the competition, the organization has no established framework by which to evaluate that recommendation. A strategic plan provides both the general direction as well as the broad parameters for the individual services. Without such, the competition for scarce capital and other resources is akin to the old-west version of the land rush—the first person or team to place a stake or lay a claim is declared the winner, with little regard to the overall effect on the organization.

Basic Elements of a Plan

Fundamentally then, the strategic plan (even if fairly rough) should be in place prior to the completion, or at least adoption, of the service line business plan. This step will save a great deal of consternation down the road. The strategic plan need not be worthy of eventual canonizing in the healthcare hall of fame for plans; good strategic plans are often readable and digestible documents rather than Tolkien-length tomes. The biggest mistake executives and planners make in crafting and drafting their strategic plans is the assemblage of mountains of marginally useful data; although it may be interesting, it is usually not all that relevant to the final goals, strategies, and measures of success. This is where many executive teams get bogged down. In a modern twist on the famous line, far too often a strategic plan is faced with "data data everywhere, and not a thought to think."

At its essence, a workable strategic plan (and to a large extent, a service line business plan) should include the following elements:

- Environmental analysis or overview (market conditions)
- Market assumptions (likely projection for three to five years)
- Critical success factors (imperative to achieve success)
- Goals for the organization (three to five years or desired time frame)
- Strategies to achieve the goals
- Measures to gauge success (achievement of goals)
- Time frames and accountability assignments

Obviously, plans can include much more, but this is a good starting point. Again, many organizations spend too much time and waste too much energy on the environmental analysis. Although analysis provides the backdrop against and within which the organizations must operate, it does not need to be all that extensive to formulate reasonable goals and sound strategies. The bulk of the time should be invested in understanding the essential achievements (critical success factors) and then crafting goals and strategies to reflect that understanding. The most elegant and sophisticated environmental analysis means nothing if the organization fails to grasp its core competencies, understand its key audiences, and execute its essential strategies.

BUSINESS PLANS FOR SERVICE LINES

The difference between a service line business plan and the strategic plan is singular focus and tactical execution. The service line plan can and should be much more targeted, whereas the strategic plan, by necessity, must be more global or high level. Consequently, the service line business line can get into more details than a strategic plan can and should involve a more thorough analysis of the operational components of the service line. The following drill-down is not intended to be an exhaustive representation of what can be contained in a service line plan, but it can serve as a rough template for such a plan.

Environmental Analysis

The environmental analysis should focus on measuring the service line vis a vis its competition (present as well as potential). It is absolutely imperative to gauge how the service line is positioned within the local or regional market. This should involve a fairly exhaustive, competitive analysis that includes qualitative (perception) as well as quantitative (actual data) measures. These two measures may call for very different strategies.

For example, Figure 8.1 is a matrix that depicts both quantitative and qualitative measures, on a relative basis, for quality for a number of hospitals in a given market. The x-axis measures perceived quality, as determined by a market research study. The y-axis is the quantitative measure that is derived from mortality and complications measures using a national database firm.

As the graph depicts, Hospital E has high perceived quality, but is actually below the other hospitals in its area for actual quality. This hospital has a clinical problem it needs to address to equal (and eventually exceed) the measured quality of its competitors. At one time, actual quality was not as relevant, but with the push for publicizing quality data, hospitals must be acutely aware of how they stack up against the competition.

On the other hand, Hospital A has a different dilemma. Its actual quality is better than most of its competitors, but its perceived quality is well below them. Hospital A's problem is one of communication, not clinical improvement. This becomes a strategy of education or promotion, rather than operational improvement. (Many hospitals, especially inner-city ones, face this very dilemma).

Figure 8.1. Perceived Versus Actual Quality

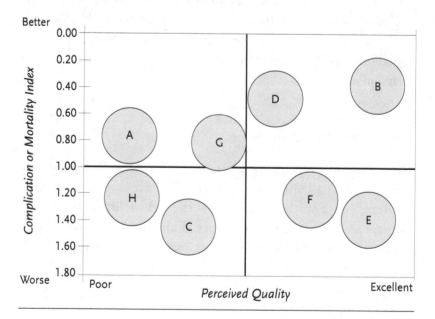

The value of having these two measures for many stakeholder groups should be evident. While this grid in Figure 8.1 is based on consumer (or potential patient) perception, the same kind of bifurcated analysis could be plotted for physicians, employers, community leaders, and even health plans. The value lies in gaining a sense of position, both perceptual as well as actual, depending on what the critical measurements tend to be.

The environmental analysis measures should closely follow the metrics identified in Chapter 4, as these will be the metrics against which the success of the service line will be gauged and the objectives will be established.

Market Assumptions

To assess the market assumptions, the management team is charged with listing those dynamics in the market that will likely have some bearing on the service line. This does not need to be an exhaustive or terribly detailed listing, but it offers a sense of what is on the horizon. Categories to consider in this analysis might include

- Other hospitals providing the service
- Niche players that have or might enter the line of business
- Physician groups that have a direct effect on the line
- Managed care plans or payers that exercise financial influence
- Government regulation or reimbursement
- Technological considerations and innovations
- Other related groups, such as complementary services, that might exert influence on this line (i.e., hospice groups for oncology)
- Local political initiative or civic actions that might have some effect

Critical Success Factors

The critical success factors are those operational components that an organization must consider and fulfill to succeed in achieving its objectives—the items within the plan that could be termed the "essentials." For example, one essential for nearly every hospital and health system would be "staffing considerations." In this category, a hospital may want to select benchmarks (e.g., peer hospital or statewide averages) for staffing ratios, vacancy rate, or turnover rate and note its relative position to the benchmarks.

For many hospitals and health systems, a certain level of profitability or financial stability would be listed as a critical success factor, as that is how they are evaluated by the governing bodies or executive teams that oversee local management. Therefore, one critical success factor might call for maintaining that certain level of profitability or margin percentage. Along that vein, cost control or operational efficiency might also qualify for most organizations in these times of limited (and diminishing) resources.

Faced with the rapid volume growth caused by an aging population and other factors, many organizations will likely list "availability of capital" as a critical success factor. The critical success considerations may involve forthright assessments of the hospital's or health system's need to maintain a certain rating in the bond market. For some facilities, "physical plant capacity" is a critical success factor because of the aging population and the increasing demand for inpatient or outpatient capacity. Given this emerging need for expanded physical capacity, many executives face the daunting issue and looming dilemma of capital allocation. In many markets, and within many board rooms, access to capital is becoming one of the biggest challenges facing senior leadership over the next five to ten years.

The list of critical success factors should be no longer than six or seven items (e.g., recruitment and retention, capital availability, quality perception, physician relationships, physical plant capacity). Narrowing the list to a manageable number (preferably no more than seven) distilling the crucial considerations down to that small number will require some effort. This is an exercise in and of itself, somewhat like prioritizing the service lines. However, first assessing the vital considerations and then narrowing the number of those factors critical to the organization's success sharpen the focus of the management team. If those critical success factors are not realized, no matter what else the organization may do (as lofty and noble as the achievements may be) it will not achieve its fundamental objectives and fulfill its core reason for existence.

Organizational Goals: Three-to-Five-year Time Frame

Once the critical success factors have been determined and listed, the next step is to list the goals or objectives for the next three to five years. These goals should be broad in terms of the organization, but definitive and qualitative enough to be measurable. Too many organizations make their goals more like platitudes than performance targets. For example, a goal like "Continue to improve the health-care within the community" sounds very admirable, but it is difficult to define and nearly impossible to measure. These kinds of goals tend to be self-fulfilling in nature, as nebulous goals are easily achieved.

It is far more productive to narrow the goal and more specifically list the target. A more progressive way to state the previous example goal would be to say, "Improve community health by bringing 15 new physicians to the market within three years." This version of the goal is easy to measure, makes it easy to hold the organization accountable, and (assuming the shortage of physicians *is* a real need) is easy to report on and likely to resonate with a number of stakeholder groups.

Examples of other goals that are somewhat broad in scope, but still quantifiable, include the following:

- Improve financial performance by increasing operating margin from 5 percent to 8 percent in two years.
- Increase market share from 35 percent to 40 percent in three years.
- Increase inpatient capacity by 30 percent in the next five years.
- Improve favorable market perception for
  a. public by 10 percent, as measured in annual community survey;
  b. physicians by 10 percent, as measured by medical staff survey;
  c. employers by 15 percent, as measured in employee round-table discussions.

Goals can be more narrowly focused to factor on major developments within a particular service line, if deemed significant enough to the entire organization. For example, two service line-oriented goals that have broad-reaching implications would be to incorporate a cardiology service line into the organizational mix and complete construction of the new cancer center.

In these instances, the nature of the goals are broad enough to affect the entire system from a capital allocation standpoint, but specific enough to require managerial attention and organizational focus at the service line level. The key thing to remember in establishing the goals is that they must have enough significance to capture the organization's imagination and enough definition to ensure that their accomplishment can be measured.

Strategies

The strategies should spell out the necessary components that will help the organization achieve its overarching goals. Some might argue that goals such as developing the cardiology service line and the new cancer center are actually strategies rather than goals, and, perhaps in a purist sense, they have a point. However, the goals of the organization should be derived as much for the motivation and momentum they produce as to satisfy an academic definition of what a "technically correct" objective is. Consequently, putting down the addition of a cardiology service line as a goal (and something that is certain to consume a great deal of management time and attention) may be of greater value than a broader-based but less definitive goal. The ultimate decision on this is up to each management team.

The important thing to remember is that strategies are the actions necessary to accomplish or achieve the objectives. For example, the "achieving market share growth" goal will likely be achieved through a number of service line extensions, service line expansions, or supporting strategies. Perhaps the oncology line needs to expand into radiation therapy, or the hospital will choose to begin offering bariatric surgery to expand the surgery service line. Such strategies will help achieve the overarching organizational objectives.

As with goals, strategies should be given specific time frames for completion. In the more detailed documents (which do not need to be shown to the board or governance bodies) that support the business plans and provide much more exhaustive information, the specific details of the action plans should be clearly defined. Although the strategy section need not be overly detailed, a document should be presented to senior management and board leadership with the type of information that deserves a great deal of attention, discussion, and frequent review. The leaders of the organization must receive this information with the clear understanding and realization that the strategies outlined will result in the accomplishment of the broad goals of the organization.

Assignments, Timelines, and Measures to Gauge Intermediate Success

Although this detailed section of the plan may not be as fascinating or intellectually stimulating as the broad goals and bold strategies, it is actually the most difficult section because it is the most demanding and least exciting. This is where the organization gets granular or detailed. Spouting off lofty goals, brilliant strategies, and crucial market factors is relatively easy, but fruition is in the details. Although these assignments, timelines, and measures will never be seen by the board (at least it is not recommended that they be shown this section), these items should be reviewed often and monitored by senior management.

This detailed section should include timelines that spell out the stages of execution and achievement as well as define who is accountable. Using the example referenced earlier of developing a cardiology service line, a timeline for completion might look something like Figure 8.2.

Although this example is not as finely detailed as a thorough plan timeline should be, it gives an idea of the key steps, each of which could have supporting detail. The detailed sections of the plan might also include guidepost measures to help management assess if the goals are being achieved and if the strategies are successful. This is often overlooked or underreported but does not diminish the value

Figure 8.2. Cardiology Service Line Timeline

Task	Start Date	Completion Date	Responsibility
1. Assign SL manager	April 2004	May 2004	Exec. Team
2. Establish a task force	May 2004	July 2004	SLM/COO
3. Complete data assessment	July 2004	Sept 2004	SLM/Task Force
4. Complete draft business plan	July 2004	Oct 2004	SLM/Task Force
5. Review/revise goals	Oct 2004	Nov 2004	Exec. Team
6. Adopt plan, execute strategy	Dec 2004	Nov 2004	SLM/Task Force
7. Evaluate successes	Dec 2005	ongoing	Exec. Team

of such periodic assessment to the eventual realization of the final objective.

Although the process may sound daunting, business plans can be the basis of a very disciplined approach to keeping the organization on track and ensuring that management is fulfilling its stewardship responsibilities to the community and to the various stakeholders.

SUMMARY

Many hospitals and health systems engage in strategic planning. However, not enough organizations take the process of planning down to the service line level where it must occur to bear the greatest fruit, and where it must most closely match the dynamics of the market.

An element of symbiosis should exist between the organization's strategic plan and its more detailed service line business plans. Whereas the strategic plan should drive the overarching direction of the hospital and health system, the business plans should support and sustain the broader goals and strategies of the strategic plans. The two levels of planning—strategic and business—should not be considered mutually exclusive or be executed independent of each other.

CHAPTER 9

Rule 7: Compete Aggressively and Strategically

THIS CHAPTER DISCUSSES the benefits of service line strategy in mounting a thorough and successful competitive effort. The role and value of the marketing function are discussed, and several characteristics and key components of the marketing orientation as applied to the service line model are provided.

COMPETITIVE POSITIONING

One of the greatest advantages of an SLM structure is what it can offer in the way of competitive positioning. As discussed in prior chapters, hospitals and health systems face increasing pressure from new entrants to the market, such as niche players with physician ownership or involvement. These new players (or pure play competitors as some have termed them) bring a level of focus and flexibility that traditional competitors (such as the health system across the country or the hospital across the street) have rarely exhibited. Consequently, whether the competition is a nimble new player or a large traditional type, SLM offers a streamlined organizational structure for competing more effectively and more decisively.

THE VALUE OF MARKETING

As mentioned at the outset of the book, the first wave of product/service line management was largely misinterpreted as merely a marketing vehicle. Consequently, this chapter is cautious in devoting too much time to marketing, as it may be once again misconstrued as the prime reason for the model. However, the fact remains that marketing, although not the only or even primary reason for SLM, is integral to the successful implementation of the concept and to the ability to aggressively compete in the changing healthcare market.

In other industries, the SL manager is often chosen from the marketing function or division. This is not necessary in healthcare, however. More often than not, the SL manager in a healthcare setting tends to be either from a clinical background or from a general administrative orientation. In either case, the SL manager will want to ensure that the marketing function plays a key role on the matrix team or the service line advisory group.

A marketing perspective is vital to successful service line implementation. Marketing expertise is crucial in the following areas:

- Market research (assessing and addressing customer wants and needs)
- Communication (vital for every service and to each audience)
- Competition (awareness of competitive maneuvers based on promotional initiatives or advertising campaigns)
- Promotion (highlighting existing services or publicizing new ones)
- Distribution (channels of distribution)
- Product development (anticipating the needs of consumers when extending the service line or expanding the customer base for services offered)

Although each of these areas warrants considerable discussion, a synopsis will suffice for our purposes.

Market Research

The application of market research, although not as often used in healthcare as in other industries, can be invaluable in assessing the value and probable outcome of new product or service line introductions. Organizations in any industry often avoid mistakes by taking the time and spending the money to conduct market research prior to launching an initiative or even promoting a service. Failure to conduct research can (and likely will) result in expensive miscalculations and embarrassing failures.

One pervasive example comes to mind, that of the major push in the late 1990s toward vertical integration with physicians. Many hospitals and health systems across the country suffered sizeable financial losses in their unsuccessful attempts to develop "integrated delivery systems" designed to provide more interface and interdependence with doctors. The initiative failed miserably and in the aftermath we now realize that the financial losses and resulting strained relations between physicians and hospital executives might have been avoided if more basic research had been conducted.

Very little was done in terms of testing the concept in a preemptive fashion with doctors and other key players in the field. The general physician sentiment at the time was, "If they (administration) had asked us about the idea, we could have told them it would not work. But they never asked."

The simple exercise of asking can produce valuable insights and even essential "epiphanies" when it comes to launching a new service or considering a new direction. Market research is especially relevant when dealing with a new model or application that involves a service or a delivery channel outside the norm.

Another example could be found in the many failed attempts at diversification in the late 1980s and early 1990s. In those heady days, some hospitals mistakenly believed that diversification initiatives—such as adding laundry services, top-flight restaurants, and catering—would succeed. Unfortunately, many of these ventures did not fare well, resulting not only in financial losses but wasted managerial time and attention as well. Yet if the initial research had been conducted with key audiences (namely prospective customers), many of the mistakes could have been minimized, if not avoided altogether.

Contrast these examples with that of a mid-size hospital system in the Southwest that was considering a foray into complementary and alternative medicine. Because this was new for the system, management decided to survey the customer base to better understand purchaser mindset and expectations. Several research sessions with the "heavy" and "moderate" users of alternative modalities proved illuminating, and the results actually ran counter to the delivery model the managers were considering.

For example, the focus group participants told the research facilitator that they desired (and expected) the alternative modalities—such as message therapy, herbal medecine, and acupuncture—to be delivered in a setting starkly different than the traditional medical environment. They wanted wood floors, live plants, and new age music in the background. Prior to the research, some of the hospital system leaders had planned to expand their existing urgent care centers and offer the alternative modalities in that setting. The research gave them a defining dose of reality before they started down a path that the customers clearly did not want; likely would not accept; and, more importantly, probably would not pay for.

Communication

In every industry and in all fields, clear and compelling communication is central to success. The healthcare industry is no exception. Yet managers within the industry have not always understood nor embraced the value of communication. Such behavior is entirely understandable, as the field of medicine (and, correspondingly, healthcare) has its roots in the "expert" model rather than the consumer-oriented framework that characterizes much of American industry. The expert or authority model, which has its origins in the military, does not follow the creed of "interactive and responsive" feedback; rather, it is based on the notion that the person in charge or control has more information at his or her disposal and does not need to enlist or solicit input from the individual receiving the direction or services.

There was a time when that model worked, especially in the healthcare field. However, society (especially in the developed world) has transformed the nature of healthcare (and medicine) dramatically. The consumer (or patient) is much more engaged and informed than ever before and is therefore more expectant, if not demanding, of interactive communication. They want more information so they can be more involved in the healthcare experience.

Nothing epitomizes this dynamic more than the rapid rise of the Internet—especially as it relates to accessing healthcare information. As one of the industry's leading observers/futurists, Jeff Goldsmith has noted, "The Internet represents the *democratization* of medicine" (Goldsmith 2001).

In that framework then, service line communication is pivotal to ultimate success. The service line manager may or may not be a good communicator, but the marketing professionals within the organization will be key to assessing the best means to reach the appropriate audiences and expend the efficient resources to achieve the determined objectives. This is yet one more reason to have the marketing staff participate actively and frequently with the service line planning and execution team.

Marketing's participation in these teams is not only essential, it will also prove invaluable to the marketing professionals. They should (and probably will) derive great benefit from the clinical experts as to the nature of the patient/consumer and the critical audiences involved in the decision process. For example, in many services such as cardiology, a consumer-only directed campaign will probably not prove productive, because the decision as to which hospital or ambulatory setting is used for the procedure or surgery still remains the decision of the cardiologist or heart-related physician. Therefore, an effective campaign for cardiology needs to include not only the consumer but also the critical doctors such as referring (primary care) physicians, internists, cardiologists, and perhaps cardiovascular surgeons.

In some markets, the health plan is still a key factor in determining which facility is used. In others, the employer (as a result of direct contracting or nationwide arrangements) will be the driving force. Marketing professionals must also examine issues such as the nature of the message, the best media for communicating, and a host of other considerations before recommending actions based on feedback and input from the other members of the service line team.

Competition

A common mistake is to replicate the strategy and approach of the competition. Sometimes this might work, but in many cases, it will be viewed as merely imitative and will usually prove largely ineffective. While what the competition is doing is extremely important to consider, it should not necessarily determine the specific direction of the communication and promotional campaign. A fair number of healthcare executives have responded reactively to their competition, rather than responding effectively and in a way that distinguishes their services as opposed to merely supporting the competition.

The notion of "first to market" has proven its validity over time. Simply stated, this is the idea that the first one to find a position in the consumer's (or key stakeholder's) mind is not easily dislodged from that position. While it does not always prove out, more often than not, first place really is the best (and by a long distance, when it comes to perceptual position).

Consequently, a marketing approach that merely imitates or just slightly deviates from an entrenched competitor's position will actually do more to support the competition than to supplant it. Therefore, the organization that comes second (or third or whatever) to the market with a service or a campaign must search diligently to find perceptual ground on which it can differentiate its services or its approach. Here again is where the application of market research can be highly effective in finding those pockets of differentiation and creating a successful campaign to capitalize on them.

Promotion

One of the greatest benefits of thorough market research is that it allows the organization to assess and determine the position of its services (or even the organization itself) in the mind of the consumer or key stakeholders. A maxim in marketing states that an individual can only be moved so far within his or her perceptual boundaries. In other words, it is difficult, if not impossible, to change people's perception more than a few degrees in a short period of time. For example, if Hospital A is widely perceived as the market leader for oncology services and Hospital B starts promoting itself as a leader in oncology, people will not shift their perceptions based simply on a promotional campaign. In fact, Hospital B will actually be fostering Hospital A's image and awareness by taking that approach. In essence, merely stating something cannot and will not dislodge someone's perceptual evaluation of an organization and its service. That takes time, substantiating data, and often personal experience.

Consequently, prior to a major educational or promotional campaign to raise awareness, assess what position the organization currently holds in the public's mind. In many cases, most people will be in the "don't know" category. This was true for a large system in Texas that conducted its research among 800 people in the metropolitan area. Over 50 percent of the people responded "don't know" in five of the six service line areas surveyed for top-of-mind awareness and general preference.

These kind of survey results usually mean that the prime perceptual position is up for grabs, given a reasonable and believable message, especially if the hospitals or health systems have a generally solid reputation overall. Back in the late 1980s, one small community hospital began billing itself as the market leader in cardiology services. This was a tactical mistake, as the competition in the area was a highly respected, tertiary provider of cardiac care. The smaller hospital would have been wiser to focus on a service line (e.g., women's services) that did not foster the concept of higher technology and greater resources (as did cardiology) and which was readily identified with the larger hospital.

Another key to promoting a service line or a particular clinical area within a hospital or health system is to ensure that the service promised and the care delivered meet the expectations created by the promotional effort. If a facility overpromises, even though it may derive a short-term benefit (from increased awareness and perhaps even additional volume), the long-range disconnect between pitch and delivery will cause more harm than good. This is especially true now as patients become much more healthcare savvy because of the Internet and the effort to develop public data report cards. People want to see what is happening, from a quality standpoint, at the facilities where they send their loved ones or that they frequent themselves. Consequently, the message delivered must be consistent with the quality available and the experience received.

Distribution

Distribution refers to "channels of distribution," or the areas where the services are provided. Historically, the main channel was the hospital campus itself, with perhaps some satellite facilities and ancillary locations. While hospitals continue to remain, at least in most areas, the hub of the acute-care delivery system, the spokes are becoming more prominent and relevant. Obviously, much more care is being delivered on an outpatient basis, and more procedures and surgeries are being conducted in ambulatory settings.

Even though there has been a major shift to outpatient services and delivery in the past two decades, in many instances the data behind the outpatient segment of the business still pale in comparison to the data of inpatient. Correspondingly, the temptation may still exist to define service lines from an inpatient basis, with not enough attention given to the outpatient segment of the service line. This strategic error can result in a failure to anticipate shifting market trends or to take advantage of significant market opportunities related to the dynamic nature of the industry.

Some very good sources exist for outpatient data that both assess the organization's position relative to its own lines and provide sound benchmark data to measure against national and regional competitors. Admittedly, these data are not as plentiful as the data for inpatient services, but they can be determined through extrapolation and estimation. Do not miss valuable opportunities just because the organization is uncomfortable with the paucity of good data for the outpatient segment of the service line.

Along with the more traditional venues for outpatient delivery, innovative and atypical venues are emerging in the industry. The push for retail medicine is emerging rapidly as a hot prospect for many systems and individual hospitals. The avenues for high-tech application of inventive approaches are also proving to be popular and effective. One example is the central coordination of ICU stations, wherein an intensivist operates somewhat like an air traffic controller in monitoring patients (possibly at several disparate locations) from one central monitor. This type of innovation offers both a means of differentiation as well as possible resource efficiency. Although each organization must assess its own readiness and need for innovative approaches, the rise of this type of creative application within the field will only intensify in the next few years.

Product Development

Many of the items described in the preceeding section could be considered areas for product development, and indeed they are. Myriad opportunities for such development exist in this field right now; so many, in fact, that some consulting firms focus solely on keeping healthcare executives apprised of the latest and greatest equipment and technology for particular service lines.

Pursuing the very latest technology can be an alluring and expensive approach, and it can prove both frustrating and financially disappointing. Many within the industry might think this critical assessment is the purview of the operational experts, but enlisting marketing professionals is strongly recommended. The marketing staff can assist in assessing not only the perceptual fit of new technology with key audiences (including physicians) but also the level of comfort and message resonance with the purchasing and consuming audiences. For example, a rural hospital with a mediocre reputation may not benefit that much by installing a DaVinci (robotic surgery technology) system, especially if it prompts the better established, more highly regarded tertiary competitor to do so.

All the components and characteristics mentioned here can be factored into the consideration and acquisition of new products or service line extensions. For example, consider market research. Some hospital executives might balk at spending a few thousand dollars for focus group research concerning a new service for an established service line. However, that dollar amount pales in comparison to the dollars likely to be expended in bringing the service on line and to the dollars at stake if the service fails to align with physician demands and consumer expectations. A good rule to remember is this: It is wiser to spend $10,000 prior to incorporating the service than it is to justify why $1 million was spent, without any testing of the waters, on a service that proved to be the medical equivalent of the Edsel.

SUMMARY

Because marketing is the functional engine behind much of America's success in industry, it is disappointing and disquieting to realize that it is not given more credence in healthcare. SLM can, however, offer healthcare organizations the framework to tap into the skills and inherent expertise of the marketing model. Although service line strategy should not be considered merely the purview of marketing, professionals within the function can use its consumer-focused, market-responsive orientation to help healthcare organizations meet their goals and become more market driven.

REFERENCE

Goldsmith, J. 2001. Speech given at the Symposium on Internet Applications, sponsored by Superior Consultants, Chicago. November.

CHAPTER 10

Rule 8: Apply the Model Throughout the Organization

THIS CHAPTER DISCUSSES how the service line management (SLM) structure, once it has proven its effectiveness with the two or three core service lines, can be applied to other service lines within the hospital or health system. The chapter also provides an important discussion on evaluating and eliminating underperforming service lines.

CREATING ADDITIONAL SERVICE LINES

Once the organization has effectively proven the SLM model with the key lines that will largely ensure its future, the framework can be used to create other service lines within the system or hospital. This is important for several reasons. First, and perhaps most important, the concept of SLM must be viewed as organizationally pervasive. Buy-in for the concept must exist at all levels and throughout all departments and functions. If this buy-in is missing, the model will never deliver its full potential. This was one of the problems with the first wave of service lines—it was viewed as the responsibility of the marketing department and did not receive the attention and cooperation that it needed and deserved to succeed.

Once the framework for SLM has been adopted and developed, it should be extended to other lines that may not be as high profile or as high margin as the two or three lines originally explored. This can and should be done gradually, following the basic steps outlined earlier in the book. The kind of metrics that were originally developed and adopted to determine the two or three core service lines should be used to identify the next one or two lines to receive the organization's attention and resources.

MISTAKES TO AVOID

Proceed incrementally. Most organizations that have been frustrated or have failed in their attempt to implement service line orientation have done so for the following reasons:

1. They have a general misunderstanding of the service line concept, believing it to be marketing centric and not organizationally pervasive.
2. They foster unrealistic expectations of how quickly the model can produce results and provide market differentiation. Service line strategy is not a quick fix; it is an elegant and effective model for focusing on the services that matter most and highlighting the areas where the organization performs best.
3. They attempted to do too much too fast. Like many similar organizations, hospitals and health systems are large and complex, which means they do not change course easily or rapidly. When implementing SLM, incremental adoption and application are more likely to be accorded realistic expectations and to achieve long-range success.

For this third reason, the emphasis, even after success has been achieved with two or three lines, should be on continued incremental implementation. High-priority service lines that will help the organization maintain its sustainability and ensure its long-range financial viability should be identified.

The process for identifying and implementing additional service lines is the same as with the first ones identified. This second wave of adoption should be easier than the first, as the pioneering work is already done. However, the organization should not assume relative ease of implementation as a viable excuse or rationale for broad-scale identification of five or six lines. The issues of political barriers, physician alignment, resource allocation, and territoriality that come with all functions and nearly all organizations will still be present. The newly identified service line managers and the supporting teams can learn much from their experienced counterparts, but they still have a hard road ahead to incorporate the planning, principles, and discipline of the service line model into their organization.

DEALING WITH MARGINALLY PRODUCING SERVICE LINES

Another valuable outcome that can (and should) emerge from service lines is the eventual streamlining of the organization. One benefit of the service line model is that it helps identify marginally producing service lines and options for dealing with such lines.

Evaluating Marginal Performance

One of the most confounding dilemmas in healthcare is what to do with marginally performing service lines. Based on their track record, healthcare executives are not particularly comfortable in this area. Yet, because of prevailing economic and other market-based conditions in healthcare, evaluating underperforming lines is one of the most vital functions a successful management team can undertake and perform.

The reasons for the seeming inability of healthcare managers to deal with marginal service line performance in this arena are understandable. First, the hospital field's origins lie in a cost-reimbursed financial structure, where paring down was not an integral component of the equation. In fact, for many decades, the approach was to beef-up services to increase the base on which reimbursement could be made. Although this changed with the implementation of prospective payment, the general mindset has been slow to follow.

Even more prevalent and pervasive than the cost-reimbursed structure of the industry is the indigenous notion that hospitals must provide all services to all people. While this is admirable, it is no longer practical or sustainable for many organizations. The world is becoming one of specialization, and healthcare is not immune to that shifting dynamic.

Hospital and health system leaders must be diligent in their managerial responsibility and community stewardship to ensure that the services their organization are providing are both valued by the market and relevant to the financial stability of the organization. For each service provided, do the revenues exceed the expenses to provide the service? If not, each executive team must ask itself, "Why are we providing this service?" The market (in whatever form that takes) is basically sending a message that the services are not worth what it is paying for them. By not providing sufficient reimbursement, the powers that be are communicating that this service does not merit the costs required to continue to offer them. In other industries, such a basic market response would be cause for immediate evaluation, subsequent transformation, and often termination of the service in question.

Obviously, in the healthcare field, this process of evaluation is a bit more complex than that, but the underlying rationale is the same. In the case of marginally performing service lines, the following questions should be asked:

- Are the organization's costs out of line, or is this a marketwide trend?
- Is the reimbursement from managed care, government, employers, or other payers appropriate (and market comparable) for these services?

- Is the current setting for the delivery of this service the optimally efficient venue?
- Has this service moved beyond its expected value equation?
- Is there opportunity for consolidation with other services or collaboration with other providers (co-opetition)?
- Are key audiences aware of the financial drag of these services on the overall economics of the organization and of the ramifications for long-term viability?
- What would be the fallout from key stakeholder groups if this service line were diminished, consolidated, or discontinued?

Admittedly, these are difficult questions and challenging issues. Nonetheless, in these turbulent and trying times, each organization should regularly ask these or similar questions about their marginal lines. Just the exercise of highlighting and then discussing marginal lines will prove illuminating for many organizations as well as beneficial for the community.

Eliminating a Service Line

Although some systems are hesitant to even begin analysis for possible elimination of service lines in fear of the reaction, elimination of a service or service line should always be one option on the table. It may not be the final determined option, but holding it out as a possibility will make the overall evaluation of the service line more forthright and objective.

For example, a not-for-profit hospital system in the South purchased three urgent care medical clinics that had been started by a doctor and a business partner. The clinics were purchased at a time when the hospital was looking to expand its outreach efforts, integrate better with the physicians, and increase its overall market share. In the first few years, the clinics, although just breaking even, proved to be a good diversification for the system, producing increased awareness and improved accessibility. However, with changes in the managed care marketplace and the area's reimbursement environment, the clinics became a money drain.

In discussions with senior leaders, the person responsible for the clinics, as well as the physician who had started them and was now acting as an advisor/consultant for the system, adamantly opposed putting a sale or closure option for the clinics on the table. By refusing to examine the worst-case scenario (at least in their minds), they were limiting their options and skewing the evaluation of the clinics' true potential and performance assessment.

As it eventually played out, when the overall system began to struggle financially, management focused on those segments of the operation that were not carrying their weight. The clinics, of course, stood out. Hastily, and not very deftly, the clinics were closed, and many of the patients and physicians involved were anything but pleased with the way the entire situation was handled.

Some people have the very misconstrued perception that by putting an option on the table it becomes a reality. In some organizations, that may be the case; but in most instances, it proves that no project is so sacred that it will not be evaluated objectively. Such a strategy also demonstrates the extent to which management is willing to constantly and meticulously scrutinize all levels of the operation in an effort to evaluate, monitor, and improve. Doing so is just good stewardship—nothing more, nothing less.

SLM Team Recommendations

Service line structure offers one of the best vehicles for assessing marginally producing lines and for determining options to deal with such areas of operation. On an individual service segment basis, the marginally performing areas can be assigned to service line managers and teams and the accountability for improving performance can be placed directly on their shoulders. For an entire service line, the organization might be wise to assign a temporary team to assess its standing, outline the options, and detail probable recommendations.

This itinerent approach to service line responsibility will provide a higher likelihood that the team members will not try to "hedge the recommendations" to ensure their continued employment. Rather they will submit candid and strategically sound recommendations to senior management based on what is best, not on what will preserve their jobs.

SUMMARY

Once the organization has successfully incorporated service lines into its operating structure and has realized initial success with the two or three core service lines identified as the highest priority, it can then move gradually and thoughtfully into identifying a limited number of other lines. This approach and application should follow the same pattern and steps as used for the inaugural lines.

Another key value of the SLM model is its ability to identify and isolate those lines that are marginal performers. This is done early in the process, when the lines are ranked based on the metrics the organization has identified as the key elements for long-term success. Once the marginal lines are identified, the organization should periodically evaluate, discuss, and determine the best option for handling these marginal performers. Options range from focusing more attention and resources on the underperforming service line to eliminating it altogether. Obviously the latter option should be carefully considered in light of the response of key stakeholders, the reaction of the community, and the ramifications for the overall organization.

The Perfect Storm (Shelter)

CERTAINLY THE HEALTHCARE industry has faced stormy weather before. The current outlook may be as dark as it has been in recent times. Healthcare costs are skyrocketing out of control. Access in care is declining. The number of uninsured is rising. Employers are becoming increasingly frustrated at their inability to get a handle on costs. Employees are paying more out of their own pockets as they question the value of the service and the viability of the model.

Sensing the collective angst among so many groups and throughout the country, politicians are weighing in every day with proposals and possible solutions. This is not quite the early 1990s, when managed care, as of yet untested, offered the hope of some resolution. And, as most pundits and professionals have noted, managed care failed to deliver. Therefore, in this day, at this time, an alarming paucity of meaningful solutions to the conundrum of dysfunctional healthcare exists.

Given all that, it is fairly reasonable to assume that within the next three to five years the industry will encounter dramatic change unlike anything we have seen since the inception of Medicare in the mid-1960s. Whether that change comes in the form of universal coverage, a single-payer system, or something more inclusive and intrusive than either of those is anyone's guess. But the current method of operation will not be in existence much longer.

Some industry experts and analysts have sized up the situation in our industry and said that all these converging pressures present a setting for the "perfect storm" in healthcare. That metaphor is not too far off when considering the challenges we face and the problems we encounter.

In that context, I close out this book with the observation that service line management (SLM), although not a panacea, is a worthy candidate for the designation of a shelter from (or during) that storm.

Under almost any scenario that we could outline or envision, service line strategy provides a fitting and flexible framework for dealing with the vicissitudes of the industry. Service line orientation enables an organization to zero in on those services that matter most to the survival and continuity of the organization. All the elements exist within the platform of SLM to stay viable under a variety of industry orientations—whether it is single payer, universal coverage, or even centralized organization (i.e., the Canadian model). Service line structure offers a focus on cost control and emphasizes quality outcomes relative to competition in the region and nation. SLM also addresses the rapidly growing trend toward consumerism.

The point is that service lines provide an elegant and streamlined structure for the next era of healthcare delivery, no matter what shape that era takes. Above all, the service line model is about flexibility and adaptability, and during periods of dramatic change these are two characteristics invaluable to any organization and to every manager. Furthermore, service line orientation is all about a focus on the key stakeholder groups—the ones that can either make your business or break your business. That kind of singular focus has always been and always will be the one trait that differentiates the blue-chip organizations from all the rest.

Consequently, if for no other reason than to get closer to the customer, the service line initiative is worth the effort and the exercise. Based on the experience and track record of countless companies in many industries, service line success will provide a very respectable return on the investment.

About the Author

E. PRESTON GEE is considered one of the leading advocates for market-driven strategies in the healthcare industry. He has been writing about and lecturing on consumer-oriented models such as service line and product line management for more than 15 years and is one of the most widely known writers on healthcare issues and trends. His last book, *7 Strategies to Improve Your Bottom Line* (Health Administration Press 2001) was on ACHE's best-seller list for both February and March of 2002.

Other books he has authored or coauthored include *Columbia/HCA: Healthcare on Overdrive*, *The For-Profit Healthcare Revolution*, and *Product Line Management: Organizing for Profitability*. In addition to his books, the author has written over 70 articles in leading industry publications, including *Modern Healthcare* and the *Journal of Healthcare Management*.

Mr. Gee is also a frequent speaker at national and regional forums on healthcare trends and strategy. He is the senior vice president of strategic planning for the St. David's Healthcare Partnership in Austin, Texas, a position he has held for more than ten years. Prior to his 17 years' experience in healthcare, he was with The Quaker Oats Company. He received his MBA from Brigham Young University in Provo, Utah, and is the 1994 recipient of *Modern Healthcare's* "Up and Comer's Award."

Another book by E. Preston Gee

7 Strategies to Improve Your Bottom Line: The Healthcare Executive's Guide

Softcover, 151 pp, 2001, ISBN 1-56793-157-X, Order code: BKCO-1127, Price: $63

With so many hospitals and healthcare organizations fighting to retain profit margins, th *book provides innovative solutions. It is not about global solutions, industry-wide opportu* *nities, or broad-reaching efforts to save healthcare. Like Stephen Covey's highly popular 7* Habits *series, Preston Gee's advice is simple and direct. Read 7* Strategies to Improve Your Bottom Line *and learn something new.*

—Russell Coile, Jr.

The book presents definitive how-to lists on initiatives such as prioritizing the most profitable product lines, maximizing the economic return of the Internet, and integra ing complementary medicine into the organization's portfolio. Along with the lists ar examples of organizations that have practiced these profitable techniques—within an outside of the healthcare industry.

Create a best-in-class organization

Competing on Excellence: Healthcare Strategies for a Consumer-Driven Marke

Alan M. Zuckerman, FACHE, FAAHC, and Russell C. Coile, Jr.

Softbound, 196 pp, December 2003, Order code:BKCO-1198, Price: $63

In today's consumer-driven marketplace, healthcare organizations gain market share b demonstrating excellence in clinical outcomes and customer service. Growing number of healthcare institutions are striving for and achieving ratings like top 100, five-star, magnet hospitals, and the 100 best places to work in America.

Competing on Excellence: Healthcare Strategies for a Consumer-Driven Market, is an executive guide to creating a best-in-class healthcare organization. Authors Alan Zuckerman and Russ Coile discuss market principles, development programs, and business strategies that will make clinical programs more successful. Learn how top provider organizations nurture cultures of excellence, provide world-class service, and develop winning relationships with physicians.

This book will give you the ideas and inspiration you need to bring your organization to a new level of excellence.

Prices are subject to change.

For quick and easy ordering, call the ACHE/HAP Order Fulfillment Center at (301) 362-6905, or order online at www.ache.org/hap.cfm.